Gilles Diederichs

My Anti-Stress Year

52 Weeks of Soothing Activities and Wellness Advice

Racehorse Publishing

First United States printing 2017 by Racehorse Publishing

Racehorse Publishing books may be purchased in bulk at special discounts for sales promotion, corporate gifts, fund-raising, or educational purposes. Special editions can also be created to specifications. For details, contact the Special Sales Department, Skyhorse Publishing, 307 West 36th Street, 11th Floor, New York, NY 10018 or info@skyhorsepublishing.com.

Racehorse Publishing™ is a pending trademark of Skyhorse Publishing, Inc.®,
a Delaware corporation.

Visit our website at www.skyhorsepublishing.com.

10 9 8 7 6 5 4 3 2 1

Library of Congress Cataloging-in-Publication Data is available on file.

Translation by François Gramet

Photography © iStockphoto
Illustrations by Laurent Stefano

Print ISBN: 978-1-63158-119-9
Ebook ISBN: 978-1-63158-120-5
Previous ISBN: 978-2-317-01709-4

Printed in Canada

Contents

Introduction

The key word of this book is harmony. *My Anti-Stress Year* renews the health book genre, giving the lion's share of its attention to physical activities and to mental and emotional peace. On the menu you will find real recipes for simple and efficient physical maintenance associated with breathing and brand-new sophrology techniques. Sophrology—the study of consciousness in harmony—is a healthcare philosophy made up of practical physical and mental exercises aimed at a prepared mind in a focused body.

Listening to your body

You feel it. Because of all the stress you are subjected to every day, your body gets tired. If your body needs to be taught to express itself clearly, you need to listen to it, lest you end up with generalized stiffness, sciatica, or even worse, low energy and incipient burnout. You need to familiarize yourself with the means by which your body expresses itself. There was a time when you were able to recover quickly, a time when an aspirin or a brisk walk was enough to dissipate tensions and aggravations. Why not learn to identify when you do too much or not enough, and be mindful of your body's alert messages? Be attentive and kind to yourself every day!

Your anti-stress program by the week

This book proposes a whole anti-stress and well-being program that you can practice anywhere, anytime, progressively, week after week. It also relies on the mental and emotional peace of awareness meditation, a recognized Taoist technique that provides a better understanding of your body's functioning so you don't "overtax" your two cerebral hemispheres, therefore causing them to work in opposition. Avoiding this exhaustion reduces the flow of parasitic thoughts that, when accumulated, make you hypersensitive and easily irritable. Meditation will bring you peace and let you tap into your energy potential while helping you develop good posture and a constant psychological immunity. As you practice, you will progressively—consciously or not—stop being a sponge, or worse. Also, by honing these important attributes of your well-being, you will elude an even worse fate: being the universal receptacle of unresolved and unclaimed problems—everybody else's plus your own!

The first four weeks are important markers, the basis of your practice: give them priority, knowing that later on you can pick and choose what appeals to you most in the program. Four weeks of solidarity are also presented here because it is important to foster exchange, discovery, and understanding of what people around you are going through—whether you know them or not. It facilitates human contact, shatters the barriers of solitude, social, and cultural aloofness and, above all, generates a community process that respects everyone's input!

What is the plan of a session?

The sessions are always subdivided in four steps:

1. My anti-stress moment: as if you had a personal coach, you will be guided to mental peace, emotional clarification, and mental support to reach a better focus on well-being and world comprehension. Meditation, breathing, behavior modification, and a good disposition are the basis of moments that will connect you to the real. These crucial wellness components will help you manage the causes of stress and, ultimately, prevent it more efficiently.

2. My art therapy moment: creative expression is an ideal mediator to reconnect with your inner child, this oft forgotten part of yourself that is all about innocence, purity, joy, and comfort. Mind Mapping©, mandalas, and abstract painting will help you get rid of the stress and frustrations that prevent you from being yourself. Every week you will also use these methods to evaluate your weaker points and your "out of sync" moments. We advise you scan the drawings included each week so you can revisit them, if needed. As for the health or well-being tips, integrate them in your daily routine!

3. My path to well-being: this is the core of the method. Its objective is the re-appropriation of your body's performance. Step by step, you will accumulate an in-depth knowledge of the way in which your body's bones and muscles work. It is important to practice at your own rhythm, without any strain. Be aware of the pain, the recurring small tensions; notice the way in which your body talks to you: specific spots rather than general tiredness, warnings of your painful forearms after a day at the computer, etc. Notice and react! Postural stretching, yoga, qigong, sophrology . . . The list is complete and original.

4. My cocooning space: common sense and easy-to-apply tips. It is obvious that your eating habits, as well as your knowledge of essential oils, physiotherapy, color therapy, and Mother Nature's incredible healing power, all collaborate toward taking control of your health. It is also very fruitful to organize workshops with family members or friends to share these ancient and economical pieces of information!

Give yourself the attention you deserve, have fun, and share!

Happiness is sweetest when shared.

Jacques Delille

My anti-stress moment

Meditation is a simple and efficient way to manage your stress by putting your inner and exterior agitations in standby mode.

Meditation brings peace to your whole person, mind, and body.

Its primary advantage is that you can practice anywhere, including at work. The objective is to teach your brain to calm down and perform well chemically (hormone distribution) and electrically (brain-muscles-nerves flux).

1. Start this first session by sitting and focusing your attention on the air coming in and out of your nostrils. This stabilizes your eyes (see drawing below) at a 45 degree angle.

2. Use stomach breathing: your stomach goes out when you inhale, in when you exhale; your back is straight; your spine is extended. Do not hesitate to sit on a meditation pillow to avoid knee or hip pain.

Important: meditate regularly to regain your inner calm.

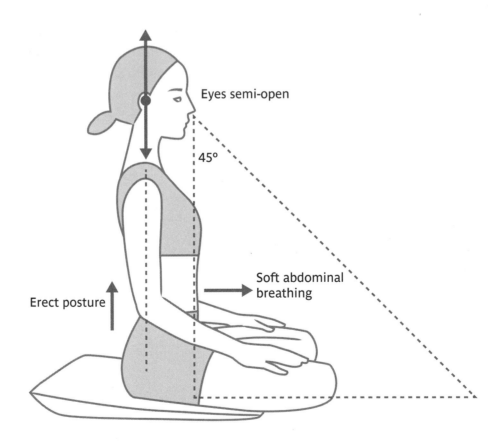

Eyes semi-open

45°

Soft abdominal breathing

Erect posture

REGULARITY ENHANCES THE BENEFITS OF EACH SESSION.

My art therapy moment

✏️ Positive coloring

◎ Perfectly symmetrical, the number 4 represents the foundation, the seat. Hence, the four-leaf clover symbolizes luck and positivity. To multiply your chances of success, use the colors that seem most dynamic to you.

◎ In a few words, indicate what you wish to realize in the near future:

. . . .
. . . .
. . . .
. . . .
. . . .
. . . .
. . . .
. . . .
. . . .
. . . .
. . . .
. . . .
. . . .
. . . .
. . . .
. . . .
. . . .
. . . .
. . . .

Meditate on this sentence:

*Luck is
the ability to grab
opportunities.*

Douglas MacArthur

Health Tip

Make your own cleanse: add one drop of rosemary essential oil to one liter of water.

My path to well-being

This year, special attention will be given to your back. Every day your hip-neck axis is taxed by multiple micro-contractions: a poor sitting position, an unbalanced backpack, a sorely tested foot arch, etc. Even if your back is muscular, you will feel points of contraction at times.

To achieve a better posture, first concentrate on your head and neck. At work, they might remain in the same position for hours or be repeatedly mobilized by nervous reflexes. Consequently, stretches should be gentle and smooth, repeated regularly during the day, rather than poorly executed for one hour.

1. Using your finger, gently push your jaw down. Repeat three times.

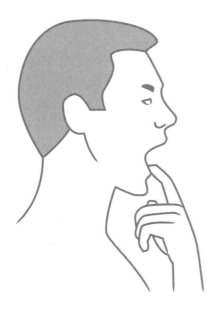

2. Mouth closed, use your fingers to gently push the left side of your jaw to the right.

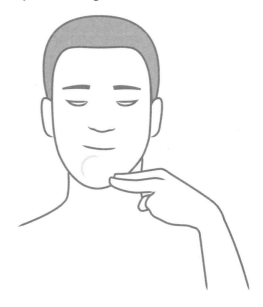

3. Fingers on the left side of your teeth, lower your jaw while pushing it to the right. Switch sides, repeating steps two and three.

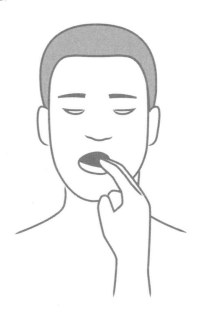

My cocooning space

Concocting massage or beauty oils, alone or with friends, makes for a relaxing moment. The massaging oil recipes below target muscular aches and pains. Don't forget to fully massage the oil into the skin and to avoid the sun immediately after!

All-purpose massaging

◎ Prepare a simple, all-purpose massage oil with lavender flowers. Keep the flowers whole and let them dry for two days, then put them in a glass jar.

◎ Fill up the jar with organic sunflower oil. Let it sit in the sun for the whole day, jar open. Bring the jar inside, close it, and let sit the whole night.

◎ Repeat for three weeks before using.

Cramps

◎ Mix 0.7 ounces of vegetable sweet almond oil, 4 drops of lavender essential oil, 3 drops of tarragon essential oil, and 2 drops of tropical basil essential oil.

Tendinitis

◎ Mix 0.7 ounces of vegetable macadamia oil, 4 drops of everlasting essential oil, 4 drops of wintergreen essential oil, and 4 drops of incense essential oil.

Muscular tear

◎ Mix 0.7 ounces of grapeseed vegetable oil, 4 drops of lemon eucalyptus essential oil, 2 drops of peppermint essential oil, and 4 drops of tropical basil essential oil.

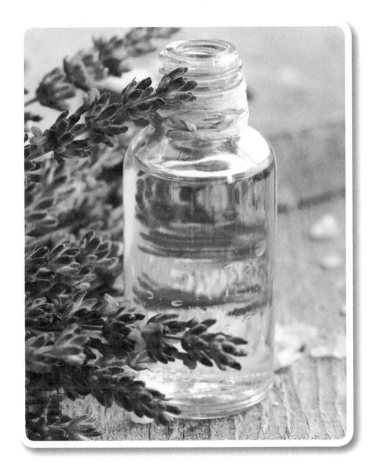

My anti-stress moment

Meditation fosters concentration. Easier said than done, though, which is why we take so many avoidance paths without even realizing it. This week's meditation session complements the work we did the first week. Practice this program every day, wherever you are (no special environment required), and your attention and concentration will improve.

1. Stop what you are doing for a few minutes and just observe what is around you. Take your pulse at the same time (see drawing). Breathe calmly so as to regulate your pulse. Perhaps you will have a multitude of quick thoughts, judgments, daydreams, tensions, and visual fatigue . . . let it all come and go, remaining focused on your pulse.

2. Concentrate on one object or one point in space and count as follows: inhale, count one; exhale, count one; inhale, two; exhale, two, and so on. This forces you to be present and pay attention to your breathing. Count to ten or more, if needed.

3. Resume observing what is around you: somebody walking by, a smell, a sound. Take mental notes. Go back to concentrating on your pulse, which is already slower and calmer. Go through the whole process once. Exhale fully and go back to your activities.

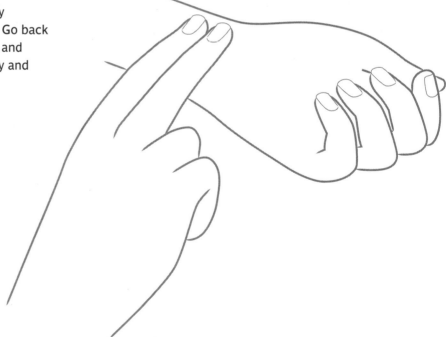

FOCUS ON YOUR PULSE, BE PRESENT IN THE "HERE AND NOW."

My art therapy moment

✏️ Offering kisses

◎ It is interesting to consider who you would like to kiss spontaneously. A kiss, generally used to show kindness or thankfulness, reveals a lot about the person who gives it. An air kiss for some, a big smooch for others, a kiss for everyone!

◎ Color each heart thinking about somebody in particular. Are there too many for the number of people you wish to give a kiss to, or not enough? This is also an indication of your affective relationships.

◎ Write the name of the person next to the heart and imagine you are giving him or her a kiss. Use this occasion to offer tenderness from afar!

◎ In a few words, describe what kissing means to you:

. . . .
. . . .
. . . .
. . . .
. . . .
. . . .
. . . .
. . . .
. . . .
. . . .
. . . .
. . . .

Meditate on this sentence:

A light heart lives long.
William Shakespeare

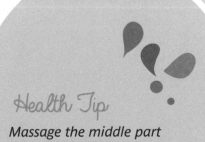

Health Tip

Massage the middle part of your torso regularly to alleviate tension and stress in your chest.

My path to well-being

Building on the back stretch we saw last week, these simple movements will maintain the flexibility of your neck and disengage your body from perturbing tensions. Breathe fully, inhaling as you stretch, exhaling as you get back to starting position.

1. Start by slightly moving your head to the left. Gently lower your chin, feel your neck muscles stretch. Repeat three times.

2. Move your head backwards and slightly to the left. Feel the stretch and your muscles working; always move gently and progressively. Repeat three times and switch sides.

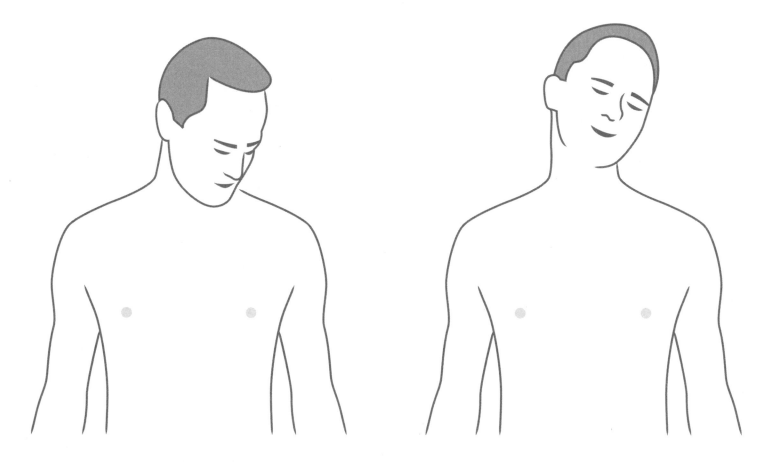

My cocooning space

The scents that surround you will concretely affect your mood and other people's disposition. Prepare a diffuser, i.e. a receptacle, like a water container, and set it near the area where you want the scented air to circulate.

◎ Air sanitizing (kitchen, bathroom, etc.): mix equal parts of lemon, mint, and eucalyptus essential oils.

◎ Welcoming effect (for guests or cold winter days): mix equal parts of lavender, orange, and cinnamon essential oils. For something more flowery mix equal parts of bergamot, juniper, and cypress essential oils.

◎ Energetic: mix equal parts of grapefruit and lavender, mint and rose, or mandarin and clove essential oils.

◎ Fresh and clean clothes closet: in a sachet, mix equal parts of citronella sprigs, dried lemon zests, and thyme twigs.

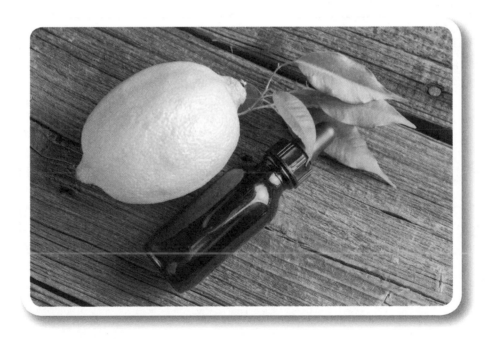

SCENTS ARE POWERFUL MOOD ENHANCERS.

My anti-stress moment

Breathing is an efficient way to let go of your stress. Breathing well is also a lifestyle. As you go about your daily activities, it is necessary to regularly stop and think about your lung capacity. Anxiety or psychological pressure is not a good enough reason for you to be in hyper- or hypo-oxygenation!

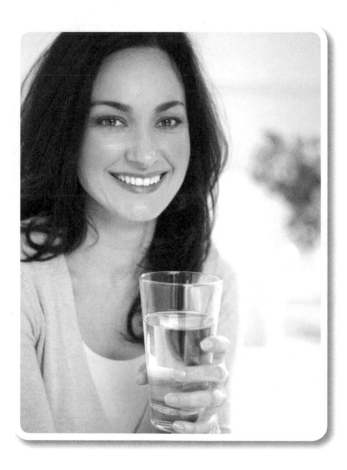

Do this quick daily routine to make sure you keep the right balance.

Every hour, take a few moments to:

◎ Drink half a glass of water.

◎ Simply put your hand on your stomach and use stomach breathing: inhale through your nose and see your abdomen expand outward, pushing your hand out. Exhale through your mouth and see your hand come back in. Repeat at least seven times. This forces you to concentrate on yourself and relax your abdominal belt, generating a proper oxygenation.

◎ Rub your hands together and, taking advantage of the heat produced, gently massage your stomach clockwise for one minute. This massages your intestines so you remain relaxed.

◎ With your thumb and your index finger, gently tug on the lobe of each ear, then on the rest of your ear. This relaxes your face, loosening your jaw.

◎ Drink the other half of your glass of water.

OXYGENATION IS A DIRECT PATH TO FEELING PEACEFUL.

My art therapy moment

✏️ **An imaginary flower**

◎ Concentrating in order to de-stress or relax is an efficient way to remain in the moment. Here is a mandala that requires precision and curvy movements. Using a palette of mostly green, white, and ivory, remain in the color harmony and use curvy strokes to follow the leaves of the mandala.

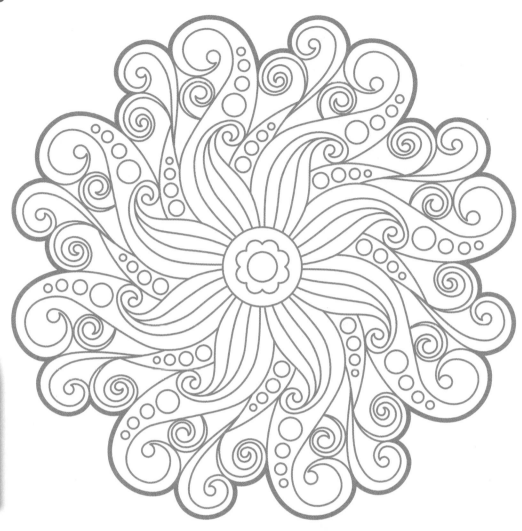

Meditate on this sentence:

'Tis a beautiful harmony when doing and saying agree.

Montaigne

◎ In a few words, note your current needs to stay in harmony:

. . . .
. . . .
. . . .
. . . .
. . . .
. . . .
. . . .
. . . .
. . . .
. . . .

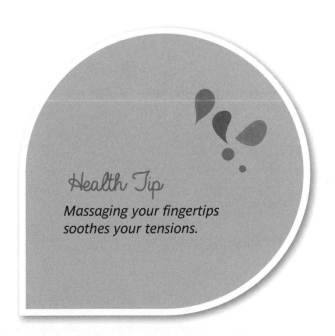

Health Tip

Massaging your fingertips soothes your tensions.

My path to well-being

This week, we continue our gentle back program. Remember 1) your practice is dependent upon how you feel and 2) ideally, stretch right after showering, so your shoulders are relaxed (massaged with lukewarm water).

1. Sit up with your back straight, right palm on your right thigh. Left palm on the right side of your head, inhale while (gently) pulling your head to the left. Stretch the right side of your nape just a little more, so you feel the muscle stretching. Slowly come back to your original position as you exhale. Repeat three times. Switch sides.

2. With your thumbs, massage the two natural cavities at the top of your nape. Head slightly lowered, gently push and let go several times.

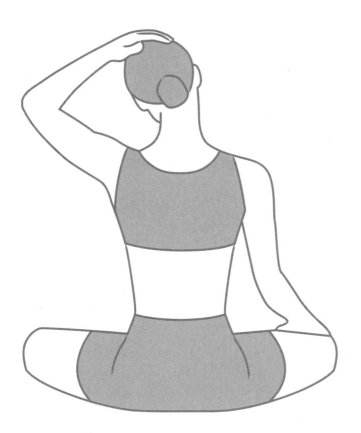

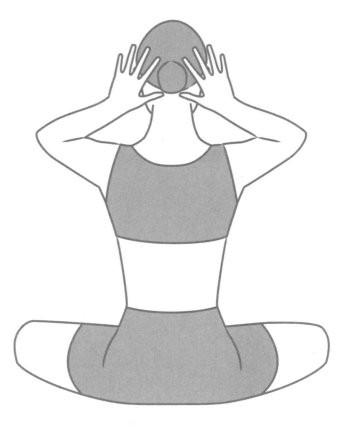

My cocooning space

Flowers have the extraordinary ability to relax. Here are a few efficient products.

Dr. Bach's flowers

◎ Get acquainted with Dr. Bach's elixirs: they are excellent emotional mediators, particularly the Rescue, otherwise known as "Rescue remedy." Apply four drops under the tongue two to three times a day to foster mental peace.

◎ Research the virtues of other remedies (some even suited for children!) and their various forms: homeopathic pellets, spray, etc.

Deva Laboratories Floral Compounds

◎ When stress is caused by obsessive ideas or fixations, or anxiety-induced tension points are preventing you from sleeping, take Floral Compound No. 2, *Nuitpaisible*, Peaceful Night. Take three drops, three times a day. Basis: chamomile, lavender, passionflower, and linden.

◎ When irritability becomes chronic, take Floral Compound No. 7 *Ressourcement*, Rejuvenation. Take three drops, three times a day. Basis: Amaranth, iris, impatient, dill herb, and mint.

◎ The line includes fifteen compounds. All are organic and very well balanced.

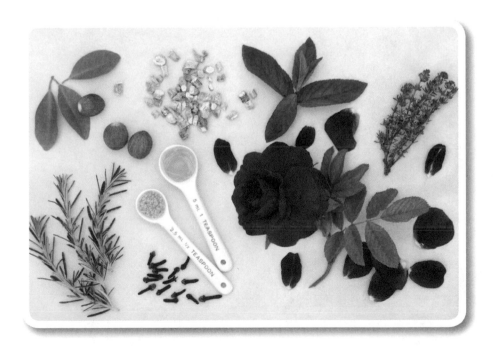

FLORAL COMPOUNDS QUICKLY MODIFY YOUR EMOTIONS.

My anti-stress moment

Silencing our mind is not as simple as it seems. During your first meditation week, you were asked to concentrate on inhaling and exhaling. Some were probably able to clear their minds, while others probably couldn't stop thinking or daydreaming.

This week, concentrate on how loud you can be. Human beings are always expressing something, particularly when silent! Becoming aware of this will allow you to better integrate into the present and accept any and all forms of life. You will identify your needs and progressively distinguish whether you are in harmony or not, which you will correct through breathing.

This is the reason why two-to-three-minute anti-stress breaks should be taken regularly during the day. Below are some tips:

◎   Take the time to interrupt what you are doing, wherever you happen to be. Get in touch with your breathing and observe people, sounds, colors, smells, etc. Stay centered on yourself; do not lose yourself in what is around you. Peace is coming.

◎   Stop where you are and listen within. Is there harmony or not? Breathe slowly, interiorize by listening to your needs (perhaps a drink, a few steps to oxygenate your blood, let thoughts pass . . .) Create a decompression chamber, then slowly go back to what you were doing.

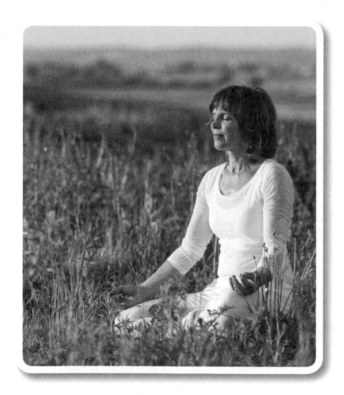

EVERY DAY, SILENTLY GET IN TOUCH WITH YOURSELF.

My art therapy moment

 Treat yourself
to an inner child moment!

Find joy in expressing your creativity. Move freely, without thinking or planning.

You need:
Big sheets of drawing paper, some adhesive tape (Scotch tape©), watercolor tubes, brushes, ice cubes, a sponge, water, and an easy-to-clean space.

◎ Create several large paper surfaces by taping a few sheets of paper together on their reverse side.

◎ Spread the first paper surface on the table. Across the top of the surface, use one color to create a horizontal stripe of paint. Use another color to create a second stripe, then a third color to create a third stripe, etc.

◎ Take an ice cube and apply it on one stripe, which will become lighter. Rinse the ice cube in the water and apply it on another color. Repeat. You can also not rinse the ice cube and use it as a coloring pencil. Get into it! Let your creative juices flow freely!

◎ On the second paper surface, apply the color by gently tapping your sponge on the paper. Rinse the sponge every time you switch color.

Thanks to this relaxing method you will reach deep harmony by concentrating on your creativity.

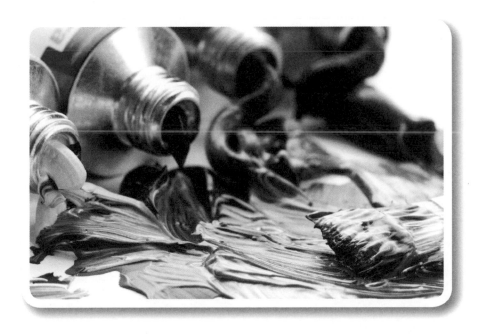

My path to well-being

For those of us who work on a computer, tensions often appear at the base of the nape. The artificially heated or cooled air we live in makes the stiffness worse and, very quickly, hinders our head movements.

Hence, the next step of our back program.

1. Back and head aligned, stretch your head backward, working the top of the nape. Breathe in as you stretch and breathe out as you come back to your original position. Repeat at least three times. Inhale through your nose and exhale while slowly lowering your chin down. Repeat three times. Associate the muscular stretch to the positive thought of relaxing and caring for the muscle.

2. Left hand on the right side of you nose, inhale while turning your head to the left, as far as possible without forcing it. Repeat three times. Switch sides.

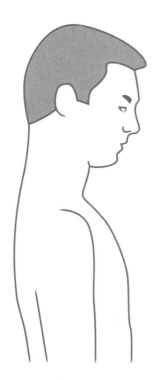

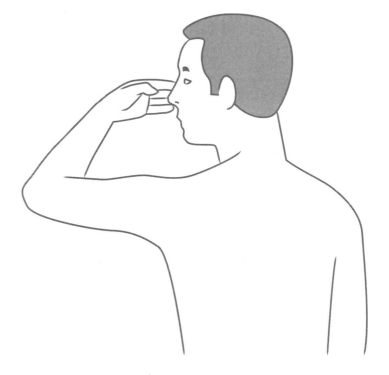

My cocooning space

Have you heard of hydrolats? They are aromatic waters—also called floral waters—that contain traces of essential oil molecules remaining after distillation. For example, as geranium is distilled, i.e. boiled in water, the steam containing the essential oils condenses, then returns to its liquid form. The essential oils are separated from the condensation water, which has been "charged" with aromatic molecules. That is a geranium hydrolat.

Hydrolats are used when essential oil would be too strong, for example in face and body creams, sensitive skin sprays, rubs, etc. Much less expensive than essential oils, hydrolats are very beneficial to the well-being of the whole family!

◎   Lavandin, tea tree, niaouli, geranium, and real lavender hydrolats can be used on a simple cotton pad as a facial cleanser.

◎   For a relaxing aromatic bath, add 3 tablespoons of geranium hydrolat while running your bath.

◎   Add some lavender hydrolat to your home cleaning products or in your iron water receptacle for a refreshing scent.

◎   In your cooking, use mint, rosemary, thyme, or cinnamon. Three teaspoons of hydrolat are enough to add flavor to a main dish or a dessert.

◎   Orange blossom hydrolat herbal tea facilitates digestion.

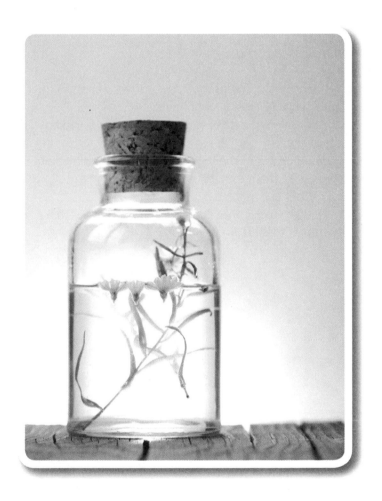

FLOWER HYDROLAT, A NATURAL SKIN CARE PRODUCT.

My anti-stress moment

When you begin to feel aggravated get into the habit of assessing the situation once a day: if your brain cannot manage, it will put itself on autopilot before a total meltdown!

Be kind, fair, and good to yourself. This implies auto-critique, not self-criticism. This is even truer if you are a parent, with daily home duties compounding your professional responsibilities.

1. Get a spiral notebook.

2. On the left page, note:

◎   Unavoidable tasks: food shopping, business report, dinner planning, difficult business meeting, etc.
◎   Possible problematic tasks: delays on a report, incipient health issues, etc.
◎   Unplanned events of the day: at the end of the day, note unexpected tasks, changes in schedule, delayed meetings, etc.

3. On the right page, note concrete solutions for each situation. Cross off when solved.

You are not a superhero, be kind to yourself! The idea is to pinpoint the recurring events. For some, it might be health issues. React on that front. For others, work might be a constant source of panic. Implement solutions at work. The objective is to better understand the problem and determine its source: lack of concentration, unproductive loss of energy, loss of touch with reality, etc. . . .

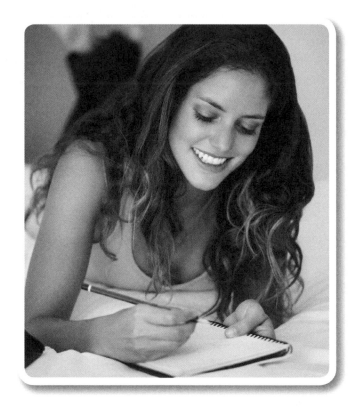

PREVENT OVERTAXING YOUR MIND BY SORTING OUT YOUR THOUGHTS AND IDEAS.

My art therapy moment

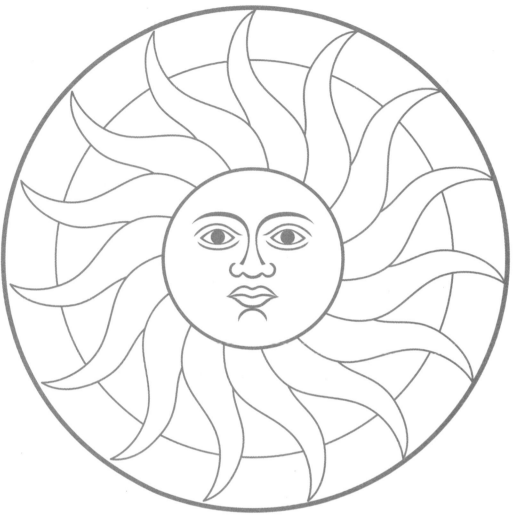

A sweet sun

◎ The sun is warm. Away from it I am cold, but too close, I burn. Emotionally calm down by coloring each ray while thinking about a different person. You might want to heat up a few, cool off others, burn someone who is aggravating you . . . let it all out!

◎ In a few words, describe how you could detach yourself from the people who seem toxic:

. . . .

. . . .

. . . .

. . . .

. . . .

. . . .

. . . .

. . . .

. . . .

. . . .

. . . .

Meditate on this sentence:

Don't let negative people steal your joy. When you lose your joy, you lose your strength.

Nelson Mandela

Health Tip

Regularly massage the natural line going from your neck to your navel. It will calm your emotions.

23

My path to well-being

Here are some simple movements to relieve stress in the top of your back:

1. Stand, right arm up, right biceps in your left hand. Stretch your back by forcing your right arm to the left. Repeat three times gently, feeling the stretch each time. Switch sides.

2. Slowly and gently, bring your left palm to your back, bending your elbow as much as you can. Do not force it. Repeat three times. Switch sides.

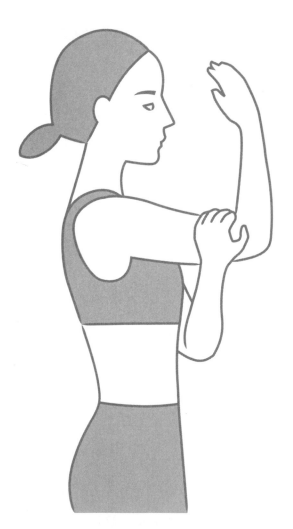

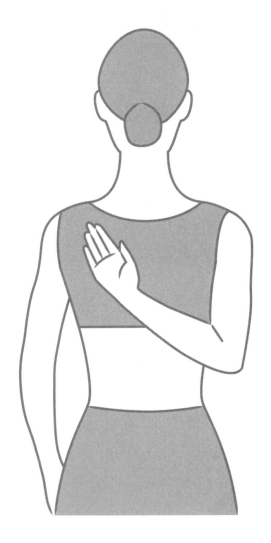

My cocooning space

All year round, sprouts are the perfect accompaniment to any dish, whether it is cooked or not. They are a good source of amino acids, excellent for the whole family, and very easy to get, since they are available in most food stores. You can also grow your own in sprouters that only require seeds and moisture (these are sold in most organic stores). Either way, they have a five-day shelf life!

Chew the sprouts well and choose them according to their virtues:

◎ **Alfalfa:** contains vitamin A (good for growth and vision).

◎ **Azuki:** contains magnesium (prevents depression, anxiety, muscular spasms, diabetes, and high blood pressure).

◎ **Broccoli:** contains vitamin C (good for the immune system).

◎ **Mungo beans:** nutritious without adding to your weight.

◎ **Green lentils:** contain vitamins A, B1, B2, B3, B6, B12, and C.

◎ **Quinoa:** rich in proteins and gluten-free.

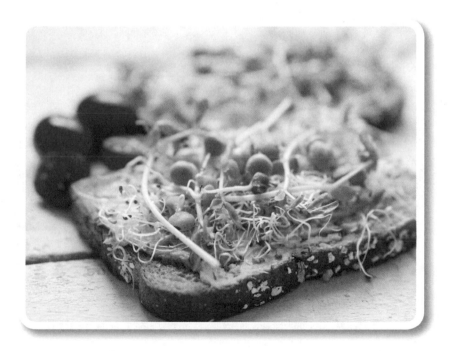

SPROUTS OFFER A VARIETY OF INDISPENSABLE NUTRIENTS.

My anti-stress moment

You can meditate outdoors while walking or sitting. The meditation session below covers both and will bring you peace quickly. Practice year-round.

1. Start with a quiet walk to reunite with nature. First, reconnect visually. Look as far as you can see. During five minutes, detail what you see without interpreting the images. Then look mid-distance and detail what you see for five minutes. Now, look thirty feet around you for five minutes, still without interpretation. You just forgot what was on your mind for fifteen minutes!

2. Then, concentrate on sounds: five minutes far away, five minutes mid-distance, and five minutes close-up, for a total of fifteen minutes of attention to sounds around you.

3. Sitting down, concentrate on the air you inhale and exhale through your nose. Let your vision and your hearing wander. Now, attuned to nature, you are receptive to many bits of information, as animals instinctively are.

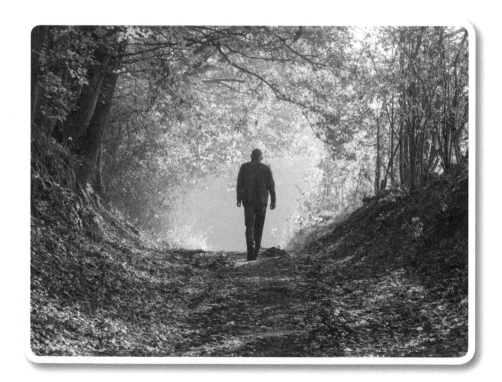

NATURE BRINGS IMMEDIATE VISUAL, OLFACTORY, AND AUDITORY BALANCE.

My art therapy moment

✏️ Emotional coloring

◎ You can express your emotions through colors. Start by coloring your anger or resentment on the lower part of the fan and progress with softer colors up to the edge. You can also draw patterns before coloring.

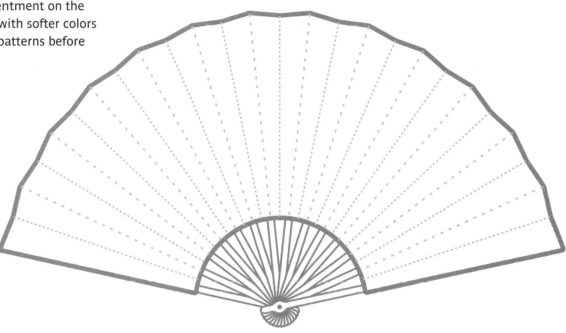

◎ In a few words, express how you could transform your resentment into positive feelings:

. . . .

. . . .

. . . .

. . . .

. . . .

Meditate on this sentence:

If you want to be loved, love and be lovable.

Benjamin Franklin

Coaching Tip

As soon as sadness looms, develop the reflex to gently rub your hands together while imagining a sun coming towards you, then smile and massage your lungs with your warm hands.

My path to well-being

Every day we carry heavy objects without flinching. Even sitting down, we move heavy books without thinking about it or impulsively contort our backs to reach too far. Gently practice the maintenance exercises below.

1. Extend your right arm, palm open towards the ceiling, while holding your elbow in your left hand; stretch your arm slowly while inhaling, then exhale while coming back to your original position. Repeat three times and switch arms.

2. Complete by folding your right arm in front of you while resting your right hand on your left shoulder. Elbow in your left hand, inhale while gently pushing your elbow to the left, stretching your shoulder muscles, then come back to your original position while exhaling. Repeat three times and switch sides.

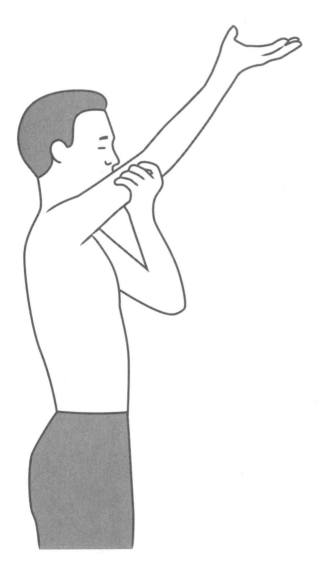

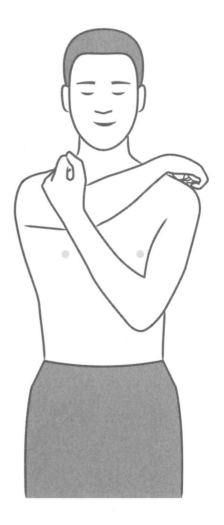

My cocooning space

 ## The anti-stress plants

Today we can use natural medicine to prevent or alleviate stress. Below is a list of readily available choices of herbal teas, capsules, or plant saps:

◎ Passionflower: calms nervous tensions, irritability, and muscular spasms.

◎ Hawthorne: regulates heart rate, aids sleep, and clears anxiety.

◎ Rhodiola rosea: reinforces the immune system and regulates nervous tensions.

◎ Orange blossom: three tablespoons of blossom flower in a chamomile herbal tea facilitates sleep.

◎ Oats: fight intellectual fatigue, particularly in equal parts with passionflower.

◎ Lemon balm: induces relaxation and remedies bloating.

◎ Ginkgo: boosts tired and irritable brain.

◎ St John's Wort: known as an antidepressant, it reduces nervous tensions and brings inner peace.

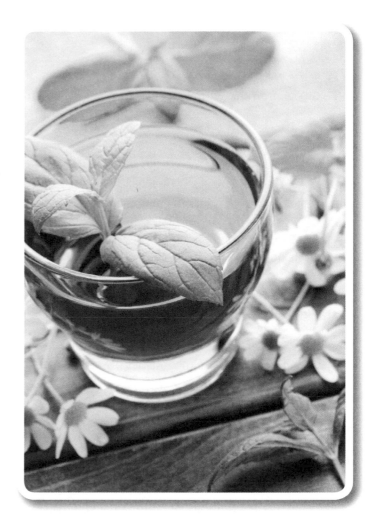

PLANTS ENHANCE YOUR WELL BEING YEAR ROUND.

My anti-stress moment

Practice relaxation regularly; twenty minutes of relaxation equals two hours of sleep! You can add to the text below with your own preferences, session after session. Be very receptive to your body's messages as you relax, since they indicate your general state—tense or not, close to stress or not. You will realize the tense areas are often the same. Focus your practice on them.

1. Get comfortable, sitting on a chair or lying on a bed.

2. Slowly close your eyes.

3. Feel the general state of your body for a few seconds.

4. Bring the information to the fore: "I am totally calm." While breathing gently, feel the calm setting in.

5. Repeat several times: "My face is relaxed." While breathing gently, feel the muscles of your face relax.

6. Repeat several times: "My arms are relaxed". While breathing gently, feel the muscles of your arms relax.

7. Repeat several times: "My legs are relaxed." While breathing gently, feel the muscles of your legs relax.

8. Repeat several times: "My whole body is relaxed." While breathing gently, feel the muscles of your whole body relax.

9. Enjoy this general state of relaxation and inner peace, then yawn and resume your activities.

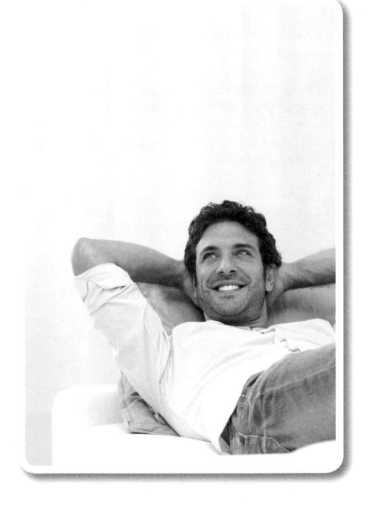

REGULAR RELAXATION SESSIONS RELIEVE YOUR STRESS.

My art therapy moment

 ## Precision and letting go

◎ Creativity moves your mental attention from a persistent idea (slightly obsessive) onto a project that literally "fills your head," i.e. becomes positively obsessive. Breathing while performing your regular activity opens a window on your inner peace. On the drawing, simply connect the dots, trace shapes, delineate zones, and then color as you see fit. Let your creativity talk and, at least at the beginning, exhale longer than you inhale.

◎ In a few words, explain what the word "oxygen" means to you:

. . . .
. . . .
. . . .
. . . .
. . . .
. . . .
. . . .
. . . .
. . . .
. . . .
. . . .
. . . .
. . . .
. . . .

Meditate on this sentence:

Caresses are as necessary to our sentimental life as leaves are to trees. Without them, love dies from its roots.

Nathaniel Hawthorne

Health Tip

Each day, if only for one minute, doodle on a piece of paper. Let the pen wander and your mind will find the way to peace.

My path to well-being

Many people have muscle or joint troubles, mostly because of repetitive movements (stiff wrists, painful forearms, carpal syndrome). If done several times a day the movements proposed below bring relief.

1. Extend your right arm and hold your right wrist with your left hand. Move your hand clockwise, then counter-clockwise. Feel your entire forearm gently working. Switch arms.

3. Fold your right forearm, fist towards your face. Simply grab your right wrist with your left fingers. Feel the movement of your right hand in either direction. Also feel the small muscles of your left hand working. Switch arms.

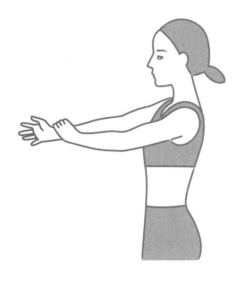

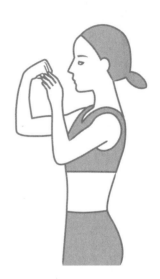

2. Right arm still extended, bring your fingers towards the floor and push your right palm towards you, gently. Repeat several times. Switch arms.

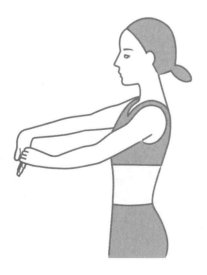

My cocooning space

Cold and flu

◎ Boil 2 cloves and ½ teaspoon of powdered cinnamon in ½ cup of water.

◎ Let brew 15 minutes. Add the juice of ½ lemon, 1 teaspoon of rum, and 1 tablespoon of honey.

◎ Drink piping hot.

Sore throat

◎ Infuse 1 cinnamon stick in a cup of boiling water for 10 minutes.

◎ Filter and add honey. You can add a pinch of powdered ginger, 3 black peppercorns, and a pinch of cumin.

◎ A licorice stick is anti-inflammatory and anti-spasmodic. Chew sparingly!

Cough

◎ Simply add one star anise into the water of your rice.

◎ It will add a light licorice taste but, more importantly, it will liquefy mucus and calm membrane inflammation.

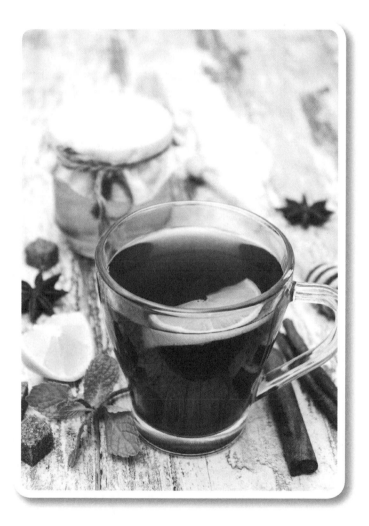

PREPARE FOR WINTER BY DRINKING SPECIFIC HERBAL TEAS IN THE FALL.

Here is a sequence of movements and breathing that will transition you into the present. Upon waking up, our first reflex is to "unfurl" our muscles, which are probably crushed by a far-from-ideal nocturnal position. Be gentle and enjoy the stretches. Set the pace and the intensity.

1. Take advantage of your bed to stretch your spine: join your hands above your head, breathe in through your nose while extending to the right; breathe out through your mouth while coming back to your original position. Breathe in through your nose while extending to the left; breathe out through the mouth while coming back to your original position. Repeat three times.

2. On the floor, lying on your back with your legs extended, use your hands to bring one knee to your stomach while inhaling; exhale as you slowly extend your leg back on the floor. Switch legs and repeat. Inhale while bringing both knees to your stomach; exhale, extending your legs back on the floor. Repeat three times.

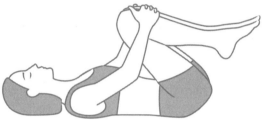

3. Sit up, using the support of a wall if necessary. Stretch your arms out while breathing in; breathe out while getting back to your original position.

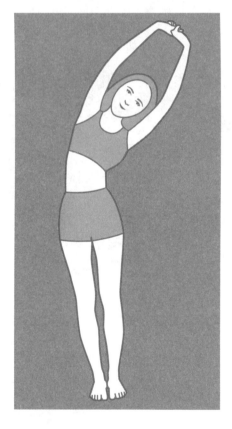

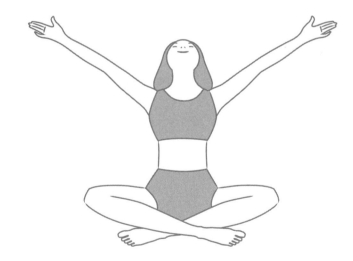

YOU ARE OFFICIALLY AWAKE. WELCOME TO THE PRESENT!

My art therapy moment

✏️ Celebration of feelings

◎ A happy mind requires daily practice: whatever happens, a human being must find ways to shine. The advantage of drawing is that you can target what you express and lose yourself in it without having to wait for the perfect circumstances. Here are two firework displays. Color them with self-indulgence, at your whim. Then draw your own and continue coloring as you immerse yourself voluntarily in the festive feeling!

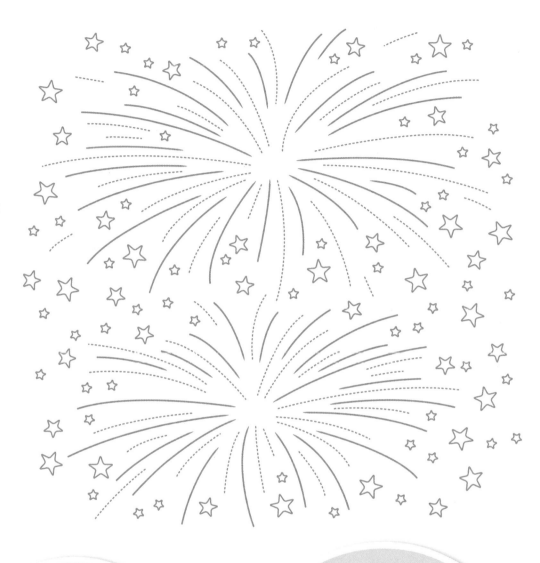

◎ In a few words, explain how you could introduce joyous feelings into your day-to-day existence:

....
....
....
....
....
....
....
....
....
....
....
....

Meditate on this sentence:

The present moment has one advantage over any other time: it is ours.

Charles Caleb Colton

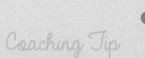

Coaching Tip

Wear dynamic colors (red, orange, yellow) when you feel a little blue. Give yourself the gift of color!

My path to well-being

Whether you are a gym rat or not, some groups of muscles are bound to be more strained than others. Simply wearing high-heeled shoes or carrying a heavy bag means that certain muscles work more than others. The following set of back exercises offers relevant and useful movements. Mentally note how your muscles feel. Exercise slowly and gently.

1. Arms extended above your head, clasp your hands together.
Inhale through your nose, let your hands lead your torso to the left. Exhale while getting back to your original position. Switch sides. Repeat three times.

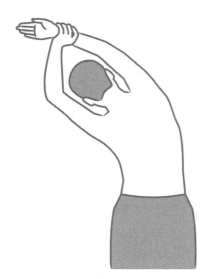

2. Sitting on the edge of a chair, exhale through your mouth while bringing your torso between your legs, trying to reach the floor with your fingers, perhaps even with the palms of your hands. Inhale while moving back up into position, forearms on your thighs.

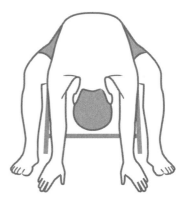

3. Variation on the previous exercise: your right hand on the floor in front of you, exhale while turning your head to the right. Go back to your original position while inhaling. Reverse sides. Repeat three times.

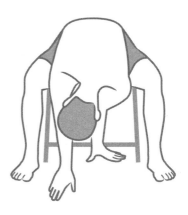

THINK ABOUT POSTURE. YOUR BACK BEARS THE BRUNT OF YOUR EXCESSES.

My cocooning space

 Appropriate daily vitamin intake is essential to remain healthy. The high vitamin recipes below are sure to add sun to your plate!

Carrot-coconut velouté

Ingredients: 2 pounds of carrots, 1 orange, 1 container of coconut milk, salt, and pepper.
◎ Shred the carrots and put them in a pot.
◎ Add the juice of one orange and the coconut milk to the carrots. Add water (1 inch above the carrots), salt, and pepper.
◎ Boil 30 minutes maximum, then purée. If too thick, add water.

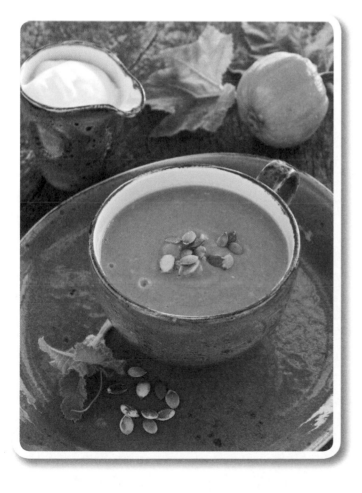

Red berries and chocolate cookies

Ingredients: 4.4 ounces of red berry muesli, 7.05 ounces of bitter cooking chocolate, 7 ounces of flour, 2 eggs, 2.8 ounces of sugar, 1 tablespoon of vanilla sugar (1 pouch), 3.5 ounces of softened butter, 0.38 ounces of baking power (1 pouch French baking powder), and parchment paper.
◎ Preheat the oven to 350 degrees F.
◎ Shave the chocolate.
◎ In a bowl, mix muesli, flour, sugar, and baking powder. Add the softened butter, the eggs, and the chocolate. Mix.
◎ Form small balls of dough. Place them on a baking sheet covered with parchment paper. Bake for 10 minutes.

Zucchinis and cashew nuts tarte Tatin

Ingredients: 3.3 pounds of zucchinis, 4 slices of unsweetened pineapple, 0.08 ounces of cashew nuts, 2 eggs, 3 tablespoons of fromage blanc (20 percent fat), 3.5 ounces of mozzarella, ½ teaspoon of powdered ginger, and 1 pizza crust.
◎ Preheat the oven to 350 degrees F
◎ Wash zucchinis, cut them into thin slices, and arrange them at the bottom of a round baking dish.
◎ Cut the pineapple into small pieces. Arrange them on the zucchinis. Spread the cashew nuts on top.
◎ Beat the eggs in the fromage blanc and add the small cubes of mozzarella and the ginger. Arrange on the zucchini preparation.
◎ Spread the pizza crust over the dish, tucking the edges in. Bake for 35 to 40 minutes.
◎ Unmold the tarte Tatin. Serve upside down.

My anti-stress moment

Often stress ends up cutting us from our feelings; it inhibits our receptors. De-stressing starts with the urge to take care of oneself.

Here is a well being path that will force you to get back in contact with your body. You must learn to close your eyes and feel each one of your movements. Be aware of every single feeling and amplify the benefits of the physical by slowly adding the emotion that well-being brings to you, the thought that you are taking care of yourself, positively. Valorize your practice and yearning to go forward!

1. Start simply standing, knees slightly bent, breathing gently through your nose. Your arms are bent, elbows against your body, palms toward your chest. Slowly exhale between your rounded lips while extending your arms forward. Then bring them back to the original position. Repeat seven times, making sure your soles are firmly anchored on the floor, like roots.

2. Jog in place for two to three minutes, feeling your heart rate progressively increase. Bend your torso while exhaling deeply. Place one palm on your stomach; feel it moving while the air is coming out of your lungs. Then use both your palms as if you were dusting off breadcrumbs on your thighs and torso.

3. Standing without moving, eyes shut, pay attention to the presence or absence of tensions in your body. Inhale and exhale, bringing a positive feeling to each part of your body. Appreciate your body!

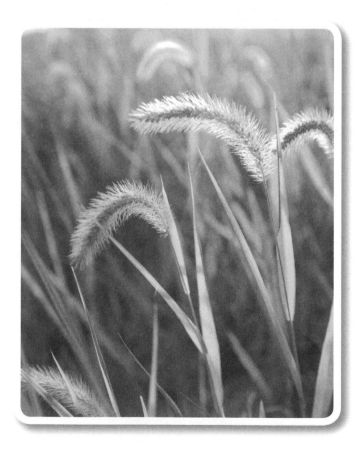

FOR A DEEPER RELEASE, LINK BREATHING TO MOVEMENT.

My art-therapy moment

✏️ The lightness of air

◎ There are days when our inner oxygen is in short supply and we would love to breathe differently. This coloring moment will help. Here are two groups of balloons taking off; they symbolize freedom. Color each balloon of the group to the left by only using the tip of your coloring pencil and only when exhaling, like in a real emergency. For the second group, breathe normally and favor light pencil strokes.

◎ In a few words, write the solutions that would help you feel less oppressed:

. . . .
. . . .
. . . .
. . . .
. . . .
. . . .
. . . .
. . . .
. . . .
. . . .
. . . .
. . . .
. . . .

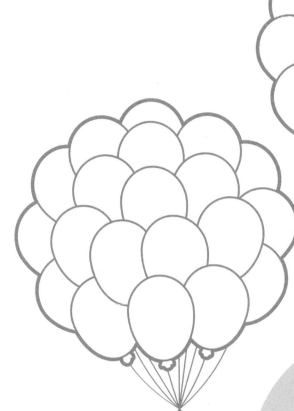

Health tip

Even when you feel nervous, make sure your posture is good, your hips are aligned, and your back is straight so you can breathe freely.

Meditate on this sentence:

Tree toppled by the wind had many branches but very few roots.

Chinese proverb

My well-being path

After sitting or standing for too long (in a group discussion for example), these gentle stretches will bring the relief necessary help to your lumbar region.

1. Cross your legs by placing your left foot in front of your right foot. Slowly lift your right arm, palm toward the floor. Inhale while stretching. Exhale as you go back to your initial position. Repeat three times on each side.

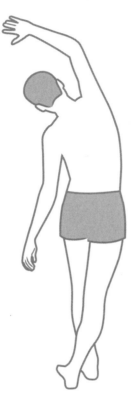

2. Feet slightly apart, gently tilt your head left and back and feel your right side stretch as you inhale. Exhale while coming back to center. Repeat three times on each side.

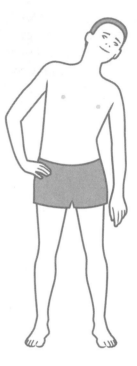

3. Prone, arms bent, elbows on the floor, inhale as you push up your torso and raise your head, nose toward the ceiling. Feel all the muscles in your torso stretch. Exhale as your bring your head back down. Repeat at least three times.

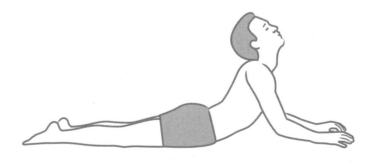

ADOPT THE RIGHT POSTURE TO SUPPORT YOUR LUMBAR REGION.

My cocooning space

Treat yourself to a music therapy session! Listen to a series of three pieces, chosen according to the following principles.

1. The first one reflects your current state (speedy, sad, harmonious, happy), a song or a piece that talks about you right at this moment (and is no longer than five minutes).

2. The second is a longer title (between seven and fifteen minutes) during which you can quietly lie without wanting to switch the channel. Feel at ease within yourself and relax completely. Make sure it is not too charged (sad or energetic); choose a pleasant and slow piece. Avoid anything that would stir too many emotions! The objective is to relax.

3. The third should be a happy title to bring you back to reality. You like it because it is positive or it makes you smile.

You just built a "sound bath": music frequencies surround you. You are acting on your current emotional state in order to feel harmonious.

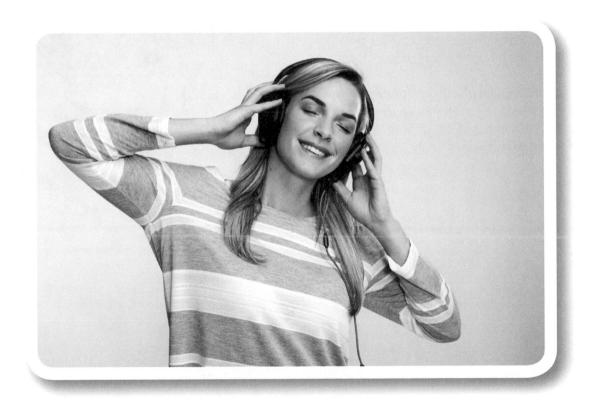

My anti-stress moment

Prevention is much easier than its alternative! Imagine the body as a powerful information receptor that the brain manages differently each day. When it is over-taxed and no natural barrier is operating, not even the immune system, the brain brews in an information fog without being able to process any of it. Aggravating! As an operating system detects overloads, the body needs regular scans to minimize its emotional surcharges and avoid frustration.

1. Sitting up, back extended or standing feet firmly planted on the floor, direct your attention to your head. Is your face tense? If so, take a few moments to warm up the palms of your hands and run them over your forehead, your cheeks, and your throat. Massage your body in order to relax. If possible, use the tip of your fingers to give yourself a gentle skull massage ending at the nape.

2. Now, concentrate on your lungs: do you have any difficulty breathing? Place your hands on your stomach, inhale and feel your stomach push out. Exhale while moving your torso forward, making sure all the air is pushed out of your lungs. Repeat several times.

3. Bend your hips mechanically forward, backward, and to each side. Rotate them clockwise, then counter-clockwise, while breathing calmly throughout the entire process.

4. Lastly, the legs. Roll the toes of your right foot up, then slowly unfurl your sole so it rests firmly on the ground. Move the thigh to the right and to the left without lifting the foot. Switch feet. Resume your regular activity.

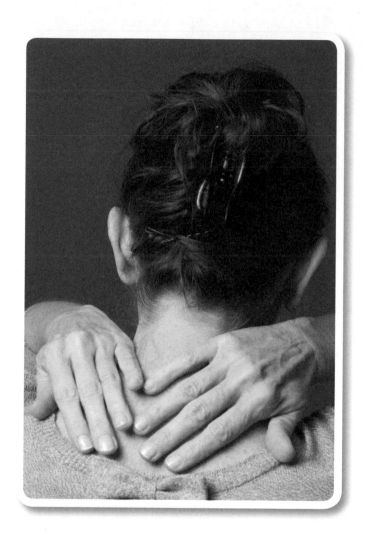

SCAN YOUR BODY ONCE A DAY.

My art therapy moment

✏️ **Making peace**

◎ Use colors to unwind. Today, only use blues (calming color) as the basis of each step of the drawing: blue and one color of your choice in the first triangle; blue and a second color for the second triangle, etc. Use blue and as many colors as your wish in the rest of the drawing, including the circles.

◎ Slowly list the synonyms of internal peace for you:

. . . .

. . . .

. . . .

. . . .

. . . .

. . . .

. . . .

. . . .

. . . .

. . . .

. . . .

. . . .

. . . .

. . . .

Meditate on this sentence:

Forgiveness is loving the person you used to be. Self-esteem is loving the person you are. Confidence is loving the person you are becoming.

Doe Zantamata

Health Tip

While you color, take time to put your elbows on your desk, touch your face and eyes with your palms, and breathe slowly to relax.

43

My path to well-being

Uncomfortable postures—standing in public transportation or sitting in waiting rooms—mostly affect your lower back. The exercises below prevent tension or inflammation and can be practiced in a limited space.

Work slowly while feeling your muscles move. Use your breath.

1. Starting from a squatting position, extend your right leg back, toes on the floor. Bend your left leg, heel up. Arms are extended, palms on the floor. Breathe in while bringing your torso on your left thigh. Exhale while coming back to squatting. Repeat three times on each side.

2. Standing, your soles firmly planted on the floor, raise your right knee and grab it with your clasped hands. While breathing in, bring your knee towards your left shoulder. Feel the stretch in your buttock muscles. Breathe out while coming back to your original position. Repeat three times on each side.

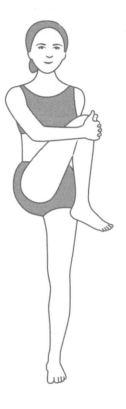

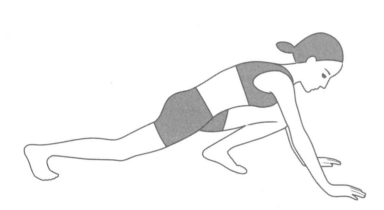

3. Lying down, bend your left knee and grab it with your clasped hands. While breathing in, bring it gently towards your torso. Feel your glutes working. Breathe out while coming back to your original position. Repeat three times on each leg.

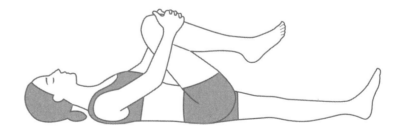

TO AVOID SCIATICA, WORK ON YOUR HIPS EVERY DAY.

My cocooning space

 The little miracle workers!

Açai

◎ The small red berries of this South American palm tree burst with antioxidants (which protect the organism against the corrosiveness of stress) and omega fatty acids-6 (muscle super-fuel.)
◎ Add them to yogurt.

Panax Ginseng

◎ The root of this ivy from China and Korea protects our body from infection, nervous shock, and physical effort.
◎ In hot lemon water, its powdered root is a blood thinner. Perfect for athletes.
◎ Refrain from using if pregnant or suffering from hypertension.

Harpagophytum

◎ This African crawler is an excellent anti-inflammatory used to cure rheumatism and articular pains.
◎ Usually comes in a capsule. Do not use if you have kidney stones.

Arnica

◎ This perennial grows in all of Europe. Excellent anti-inflammatory. Also very useful for sprained muscles, tendinitis, and muscular pain.

Queen of the meadows or Meadowsweet

◎ This perennial wildflower is used as herbal tea for its diuretic proprieties. Excellent as an anti-inflammatory or to eliminate blood toxins after physical training.

Horsetail (Equisetum)

◎ A real silica concentrate, horsetail contributes to body remineralization and speeds up bone strengthening after an accident.
◎ Sold in capsules or as an herbal tea.

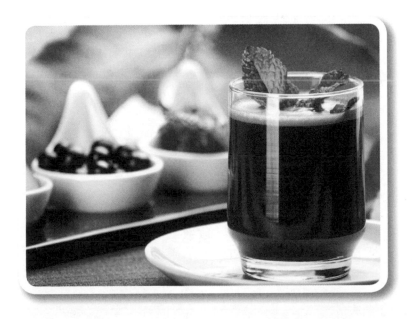

Group exchange

Group exchanges can be organized at the office and are an original way to enhance professional relations and have people converge around an employee-driven project.

Through your HR director, ask that employees be granted some time to post ideas for a group exchange on a dedicated billboard (can be done during a twenty-minute break or right before lunch time, for example.) On your end, offer this flash relaxation session. Participants can personalize it, knowing that the written description of the session will be made available to them.

Flash relaxation

1. Sitting, bring your attention to the various contact points of your body (back, glutes, legs, feet). Breathe calmly.

2. Concentrate on your feet. Do they feel cold or hot? Do you feel a general tension? Breathe in and out while concentrating on this tension with the will to make it disappear progressively. Go up your legs. Are your shins relaxed or tense?

3. Your thighs, are they light or heavy? What is your sensation?

4. Is your back relaxed? Are there areas of tension? Where?

5. Front of your body. Breathe calmly. Be receptive to the various sensations in your thorax. Any tense area? Mentally breathe in and breathe out on it, bringing it softness, relaxation.

6. Now your stomach: is it hot or cold? Your arms? Be aware of every sensation, pleasant or not.

7. On to your head. Sensations on the face, mouth, cheeks, forefront. How is the inside of your head: tense or relaxed?

8. End by imagining that when you breathe, air comes in through your feet, runs along your body and leaves through your head. Reverse when exhaling.

MAKING WELL-BEING THE THEME OF A GROUP EXCHANGE BENEFITS EACH PARTICIPANT.

Group Creativity

With family, friends, or within an association, organize a group exchange moment using the mandala below.

◎ Make sure you have enough square copies for each participant. Install the mandala on a dedicated wall.

◎ Collectively agree on the main theme of the group exchange. Inscribe it in the center of the mandala (in no more than five squares). Example: Group action.

◎ Each participant contributes a word about the main theme. First word goes in the first external square, getting closer to the center.

◎ The participants generate a list of ideas on the collectively chosen topic. Everyone benefits, since each idea is transmitted for implementation to the person in charge.

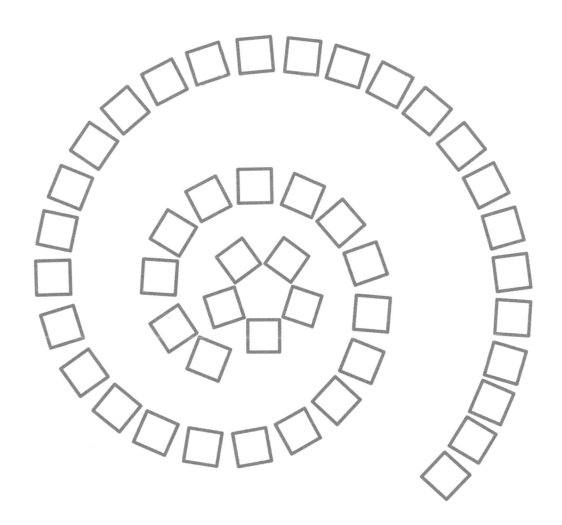

Art Therapy Collective

Each essential oil has its specificity and virtues. Here is how to conduct an introductory workshop on easily available essential oils recommended for everyday aches and pains.

The participants are sitting in a circle. The leader of the workshop sits at the focal point of the circle with a basket of oils and several swaths of clean cloth. S/he puts two drops of the first oil on a swath and announces the possible benefits. Each participant comes up to smell the oil and guess its name. Only relaxation and/or concentration enhancing oils are presented. Word of caution: pregnant women and babies should not use essential oils!

◎   English lavender (*Lavandula angustifolia*): its calming virtues are beneficial to the mind.

◎   Lemon (*Citrus limon*): a tonic used as a concentration and mind booster. The oil is also purifying.

◎   Concentration enhancing mix: equal portions of rosemary (*Rosmarinus officinalis*) and tropical basil (*Ocimum basilicum*) essential oils.

◎   Long-term mental clarity: diffuse a mix of rosemary (Rosmarinus officinalis) and clary sage (*Salvia Sclarea*) essential oil with lemon (*Citrus limon*) essence.

◎   Bergamot orange (*Citrus aurantium bergamia*): essential oil that will delicately relax you and promote concentration.

◎   Peacefulness: mix equal parts of chamomile (*Chamaemelum nobile*) and English lavender (*Lavandula angustifolia*) essential oils.

◎   Clearing an emotionally charged atmosphere: mix lemon (*Citrus limon*) with naouli (*Melaleuce quinquenervia*) essential oils.

◎   Zen attitude: mix equal parts of geranium (*Pelargonium graveolens*) essential oil and grapefruit (*Citrus paradise*) essence.

DISCOVER THE SPECIFICITY OF EACH ESSENTIAL OIL.

My anti-stress moment

Wasting time is a source of stress: looking for my keys, trying to remember to go to the pharmacy, etc. Often the reason is a failing memory, which in turn causes a loss of self-confidence and contributes to preventable stress.

Below is a general checklist of easy to implement solutions:

◎ By the main door of your home, put a trinket basket in which you drop your keys, your wallet, etc.

◎ On your desk, place the mail (new or not yet archived) and your agenda, etc.

◎ On your computer, create a file with your personal tasks (house cleaning, searches on Internet, reservations or information for your vacations, etc.)

◎ On the fridge or a location evident for everybody to see, place a family agenda (children's activities, shopping . . .), family member's timetable, etc.

Exercise

For each of the four solutions proposed, repeat the following for twenty-one days. Sitting down, breathe calmly. Close your eyes and visualize yourself (for the first solution) dropping off your keys and wallet in the trinket basket. Then bring your two index fingers together and think intently: "Each day, I drop my keys, I drop my wallet (list each object you have decided to drop) in the trinket basket. When you feel you are forgetting something or are looking for something, bring your two index fingers together and recall your visualization. Simple and efficient, this works because your brain registers the image as a successful action, not a stressful moment. Your brain is a fantastic hard drive!

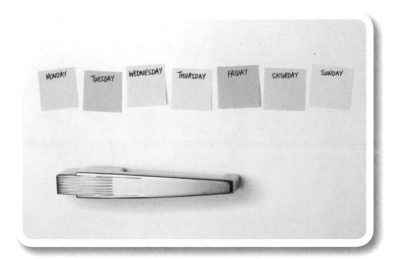

BEING SYSTEMATIC FREES YOU FROM CONSTRAINT.

My art therapy moment

✏️ Family Mandala

◎ In the center of the circle, put a picture of yourself or simply write your name. Based on your mood, position the people you interact with regularly according to how close you feel to them. Finally, link these people to you by describing the type of relation that truly exists between you, the problems or the joys, the possible evolution of the relationship. Fun, relaxing, and very telling.

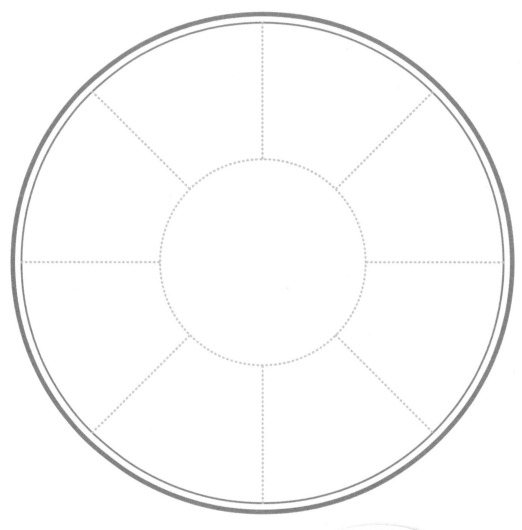

◎ In a few words, try to clarify your thoughts after having completed this mandala:

. . . .
. . . .
. . . .
. . . .
. . . .
. . . .
. . . .
. . . .
. . . .
. . . .
. . . .
. . . .
. . . .
. . . .
. . . .

Meditate on this sentence:

Turn toward the sun, the shadow will be behind you.

Maori proverb

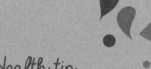

Health tip

Alternate rubbing your neck with your hands and stretching your head back.

50

My path to well-being

When walking a short distance or waiting/talking on the sidewalk, people's posture is not the best. This causes leg pains or even cramps, particularly in the feet. Here are a few leg stretches to combat them!

1. Leaning on a wall, extend your right leg backwards, toenails touching the floor. Put some weight on your toes. Feel the lower leg working.

2. Roll your feet to each side to work on each toe. Switch legs.

3. Still leaning on the wall, extend your right leg backwards, keeping your foot on the floor. Bend your arms so your body goes forward and gently stretch the back of your right leg. Switch legs.

4. Sitting down, bend one knee in. Take a towel in your hand, pass it over the sole of your extended leg and, by gently moving the towel from one side to the other, activate your leg and ankle muscles. Take a rest lying down. Switch legs.

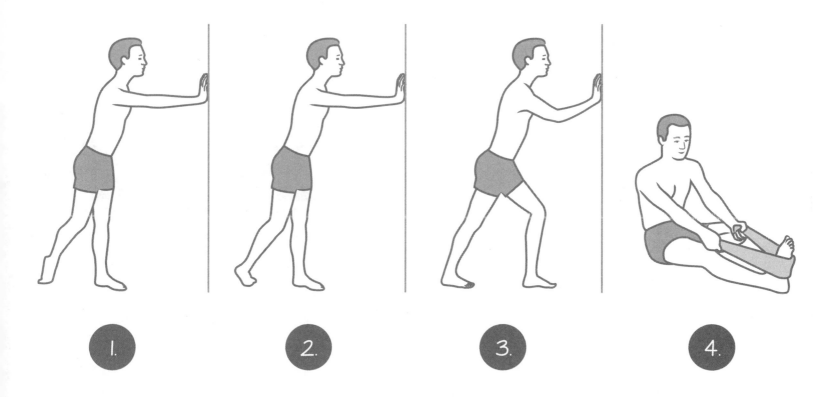

1.   2.   3.   4.

My cocooning space

Tips to monitor your weight are always useful, especially when they are sensible and easy to implement!

◎   Take long, hot showers! Finish using cold water to stimulate blood circulation and eliminate toxins.

◎   Make a point of massaging your hips, your stomach, your buttocks, and your thighs with a rubber nub brush, which will foster better water circulation in your body. Additionally, massage the same area with an anti-cellulitis cream containing coffee to smooth your skin.

◎   Regarding your food intake, citrus (lemon, orange, grapefruit) naturally enhances the immune system. The more your body responds favorably to fatigue/anxiety management, the less stress you will carry with you.

◎   Chew your food longer: the nutrients are better absorbed and you end up eating less.

◎   Boost your digestive and immune systems: every three months, take one teaspoon of activated carbon dissolved in water for seven days. Follow with one probiotic dose for seven days to restore your gut flora.

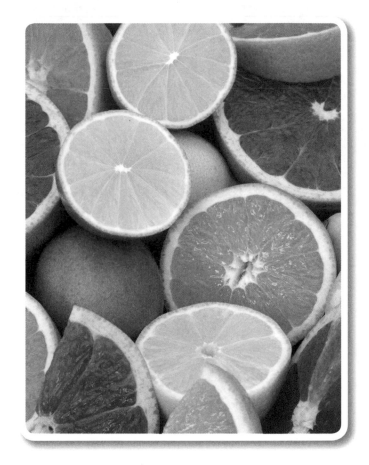

BE PROACTIVE IN MAINTAINING YOUR SHAPE AND WEIGHT.

My anti-stress moment

To fight stress concretely, put yourself in a positive spiral.

Mind your words

◎   Every hour pay close attention to the way you express yourself. Are the words precise or out of line, aggressive?
◎   Is your tone of voice adequate to the situation? What type of words did you use?
◎   Be mindful of what you sound like, how you use humor. Step back and check whether you tease more than you encourage. Simple modifications in your communication style might prevent difficult and therefore stressful comebacks.

Positive visualization

◎   In the long term, what could you do to concretely make a positive attitude viable?
◎   Before falling asleep, visualize yourself at work, in a peaceful and supportive atmosphere. The night will amplify your resolve to adopt and put in place a positive and stress-free behavior.

Making it conscious

◎   At the end of the day, take five minutes to note the moments when you felt positive, and the concrete results: participating in discussion, improving contacts with colleagues, giving positive advice, etc. Praise yourself.
◎   Now note the occasions when you could have been more positive and what could have been implemented. Encourage your desire to do better without undercutting yourself!

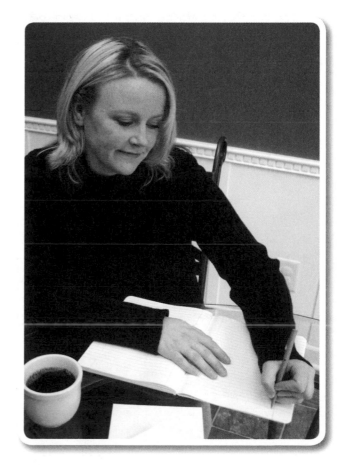

My art therapy moment

✎ Nature as a mandala

◎ Cooking will indeed bring you joy and a wish to share. The creative and meditative act of baking a fruit tart in the shape of a mandala requires you to associate colors, tastes, and shapes. We offer one example, but feel free to create your own tart using seasonal fruits. Then share your mandala with a person close to you.

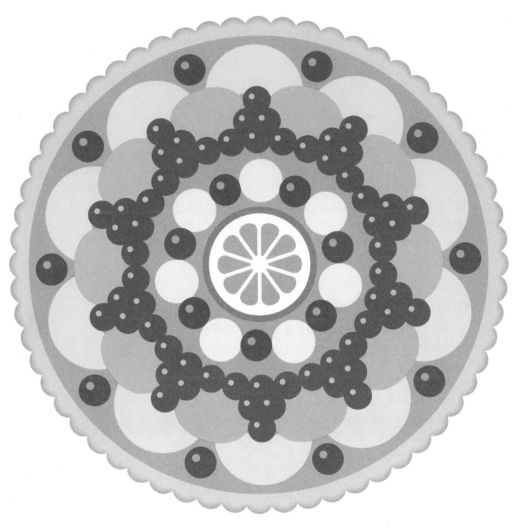

Meditate on this sentence:

In love as in cooking, what is done quickly is done poorly!

Anonymous

◎ In a few words, describe how you felt while making this recipe:

. . . .

. . . .

. . . .

. . . .

. . . .

. . . .

. . . .

. . . .

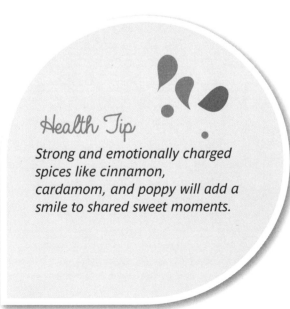

Health Tip

Strong and emotionally charged spices like cinnamon, cardamom, and poppy will add a smile to shared sweet moments.

My path to well-being

Muscled feet and supple ankles contribute to the right positioning of your arch, and therefore to a straight and reactive spine!

1. Sitting, the arch of your right foot firmly planted on the floor, use your left index to bring your big toe up. Feel your arch working. Be very gentle.

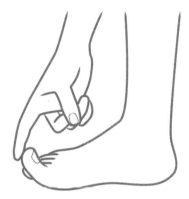

3. Very gently, stretch the four toes of your right foot toward you and then stretch your big toe.

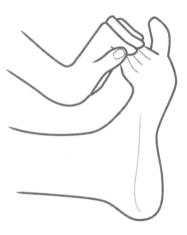

2. Repeat on the little toe of your right foot several times. Switch feet.

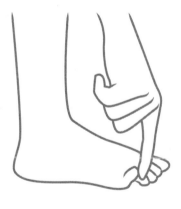

4. Stretch the four toes of your right foot away from you and then stretch your big toe. Switch feet. Rub your two feet with the palm of your hands to warm them up.

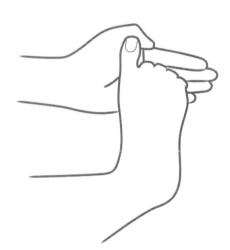

My cocooning space

Cocooning also means you can elect to do what you want for a weekend. For example:

◎ I read a magazine or a book in which I lose myself and my tired brain.

◎ I cook what nurtures my soul and my heart.

◎ I decide to take a phone call, or not.

◎ I don't do anything that looks unpleasant.

◎ I take a little time to write down everything that is on my mind.

◎ I choose or impose, if necessary, a movie or a television show.

◎ I take a nap or stay in bed as long as I want.

◎ I monopolize the bathroom for an exfoliation session.

◎ I treat myself to an essential oil foot reflexology session.

◎ I taste some teas with hard to pronounce names and ancient virtues.

◎ I treat myself to breakfast alone in an upscale restaurant.

◎ I treat myself to a peaceful meditation session outdoors.

◎ I let my eyes wander in the colors and depth of the scenery.

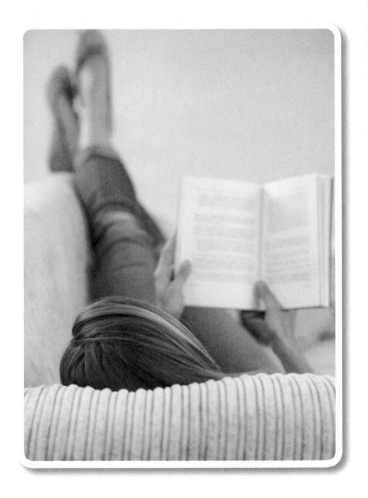

TREATING YOURSELF IS A WAY TO DEAL WITH STRESS.

My anti-stress moment

It bears repeating: if you don't pay constant attention to your posture, you quickly and unconsciously compensate with poor movements and become more prone to stress. It is even truer for people who are standing all day or constantly going from a standing to a sitting position, or vice versa.

Here are a few physical maintenance exercises to practice regularly for a few minutes:

1. Raise your arms while inhaling and bring them down while exhaling. Repeat ten times.

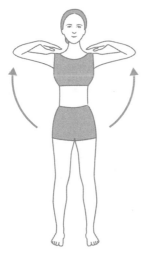

2. Repeat elbows bent ten times.

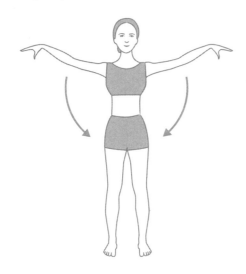

3. On all fours, inhale while pushing your stomach to arch your back. Exhale while relaxing. Repeat ten times.

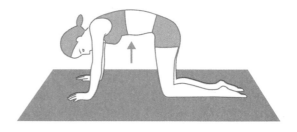

4. Lying on your back, slowly bring your knees to your stomach. Put your hands on the back of your head to bring it up gently. Repeat ten times.

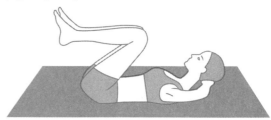

5. Lying on your stomach, legs stretched, use your toes and your arms to stretch your body. Come back to the floor and relax.

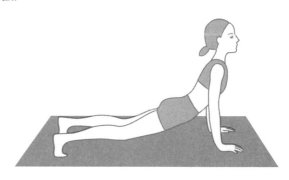

My art therapy moment

 ## Drawing as an escape

◎ We all welcome a change of environment. Let your mind wander in colors that conjure up beach and relaxation.

◎ In a few words, describe your need for a nurturing, colorful world:

. . . .
. . . .
. . . .
. . . .
. . . .
. . . .
. . . .
. . . .
. . . .
. . . .
. . . .
. . . .
. . . .
. . . .
. . . .
. . . .
. . . .
. . . .
. . . .
. . . .

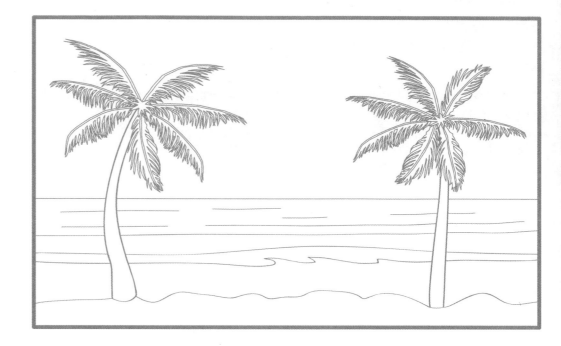

Meditate on this sentence:

The first and best victory is to conquer yourself.

Plato

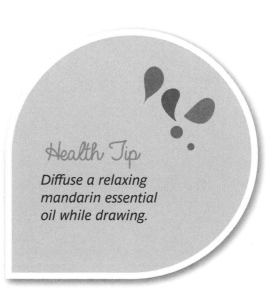

Health Tip

Diffuse a relaxing mandarin essential oil while drawing.

My path to well-being

Voluntarily concentrating on sounds can directly modify your mental state. This is the function of mantras: you are going to create yours, repeating it mentally so it creates space and relaxation within you.

◎   Take a piece of paper and a pencil. Calmly breathe and concentrate on writing words that bring escape, oxygen, peace, or joy. For example: a blue sky, a smile, a sunny beach day, laughter, fruit salads, etc.

◎   Write one or two sentences containing these words, extremely simple sentences so you will memorize them easily: Margo's smile is like a blue sky, and Julian's laughter reminds me of a sunny beach day.

◎   Lying on the floor, eyes closed and arms along your sides, breathe slowly, then repeat your personal mantras. Without changing the mood, visualize each element: the smile, the laughter, etc. Let space and joy grow in you. Enjoy the moment and take the time to benefit from this positive wave.

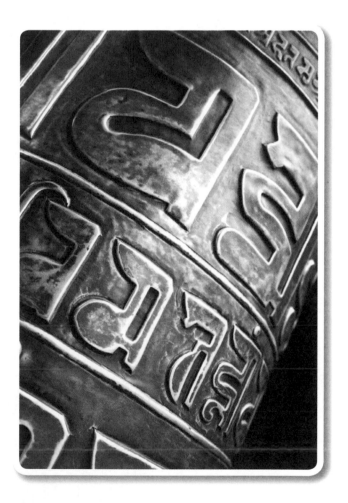

LET A JOY MANTRA CONSCIOUSLY CHANGE YOUR MOOD.

My cocooning space

Wild nettle is finally respected again. Here are several ways in which you can use it and enjoy it. Use gloves to harvest it!

 ## Shampoo

◎ Boil 3.5 ounces of nettles in 1 liter of water for 15 minutes. Mix and store in a bottle. Energetically massage your scalp with one glass of the mixture to revitalize your hair.

 ## Herbal tea

◎ Boil a handful of nettles in 2 liters of water. Throw away the plants, add one teaspoon of honey. Drink a cup a day for one week. Nettles contain a lot of iron. This herbal tea is ideal during menstruation and in case of prostate problems.

 ## Nettle quiche

◎ Beat three eggs with 3.5 ounces of flour, 17 ounces of milk, 2.5 ounces of grated Gruyere, and 3.5 ounces of nettles. Cover a tart dish with puff pastry. Transfer the egg mixture. Bake 40 minutes at 355 degrees F.

Nettle liquid manure

◎ A natural and anti-parasite fertilizer, nettle manure maintains your garden organically. Roughly cut 1.1 pounds of nettles and add to 10 liters of water. Allow to ferment in a closed container. Within 10 to 15 days the fermentation bubbles disappear. Filter the preparation and keep in opaque glass jars. Pour the manure around your plants each season or spray it on the leaves to prevent parasites. The manure is very strong so you might have to dilute it. See your local specialist.

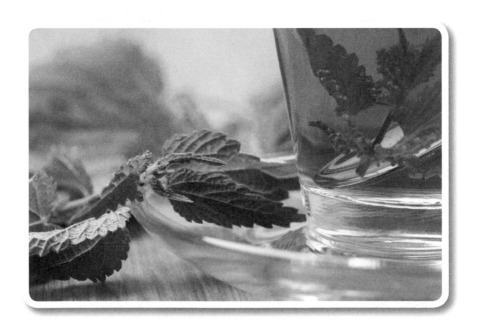

My anti-stress moment

Music therapy uses a musical message that surrounds you with targeted sounds. Their frequency acts on our cells, bringing peace or energy. This is why, on any given day, we elect to listen to a type of music rather than another. Anti-stress music is not spacy. It is a music that modifies our mental alertness, which, under stress, tries to establish total control, straining the body in the process.

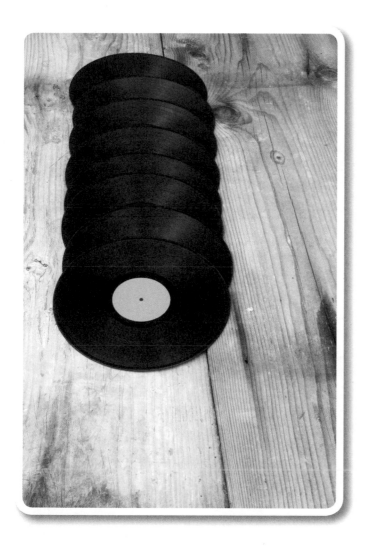

Here is how to use music to get rid of stress:

1. Lying down, position your soles four inches away from your speakers. Our soles host numerous reflexology points as well as a "suction" Chakra, a receptor of telluric energy.
Play music that links you to the earth: soft drums, low frequency instruments like the cello, a cappella male voices. Concentrate on your soles, as if the speakers were your own feet. Let the sound message flow in.

2. Place speakers on each side of your body, close to your ribs.
Choose a soft, surrounding, nurturing music: lighter sounds, no strong drums or high pitch percussions (like jingle bells). Feel the sound waves go through your body.

3. Finish with the speakers at the top of your head and play a piece with higher frequency instruments like the harp or the oboe. Listen quietly.

You have harmonized the three levels of your body. Do not hesitate to also use nature sounds like waves, cascades, wind, forests, birds, streams, etc.

MUSIC DIRECTLY AFFECTS YOUR EMOTIONS. USE IT.

My art therapy moment

✏️ De-stressing the yin and the yang

◎ Your energy is galvanized by the combination of two energies called the yin (feminine energy) and the yang (masculine energy). To be in harmony, your body needs to create a balance between these two forces. Start by coloring the central Tao sign in black and white; then use soft colors as you work your way outwards.

◎ In a few words, note your desire of harmony, joyous rebirth:

. . . .
. . . .
. . . .
. . . .
. . . .
. . . .
. . . .
. . . .
. . . .
. . . .
. . . .
. . . .
. . . .
. . . .
. . . .

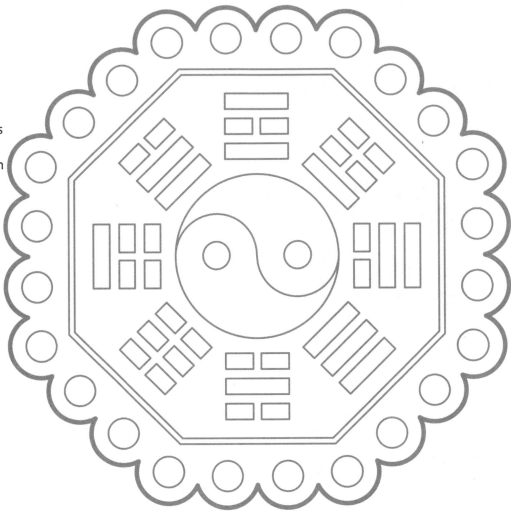

Meditate on this sentence:

'Tis a beautiful harmony when doing and saying agree.

Montaigne

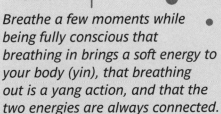

Health Tip

Breathe a few moments while being fully conscious that breathing in brings a soft energy to your body (yin), that breathing out is a yang action, and that the two energies are always connected.

My path to well-being

Below is a path to breathing that you can memorize. It is simple, efficient, and will be with you every day to maintain your mental and physical balance.

In the morning

◎ With your thumb, block your right nostril. Block your left nostril with your index. Lift your thumb and exhale.

◎ Inhale through your right nostril, left nostril still blocked with your index. Exhale through your left nostril while blocking your right nostril with your thumb.

◎ Inhale through the left nostril, right nostril still blocked with your thumb. Exhale through your right nostril while blocking the left nostril with the index, etc.

◎ Repeat for three minutes. You are working directly on the yin and the yang meridians, getting a deep oxygenation. It is an excellent way to de-stress and reach mental and emotional balance.

At noon

◎ Position your ten fingers on the natural line between your breasts. Breathe in, inflating your stomach, then your chest, while stimulating the center of your chest by pushing and letting go several times.

◎ When you are finished breathing in, let go of your fingers and slowly exhale, if possible moving the torso forward. This stimulates your heart and relaxes your intestines.

◎ Repeat ten times.

In the evening

◎ Lying down for a moment, inhale through the nose to inflate your stomach, your lungs, and lift your shoulders; then breathe out and relax the shoulders, lungs, stomach.

◎ Repeat ten times to get rid of the day's stress.

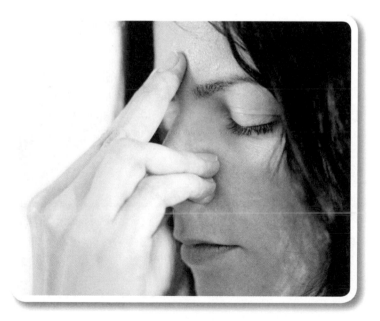

YOUR BREATHING DIRECTLY REGULATES YOUR STRESS.

My cocooning space

 There is more to taking care of your body than a daily shower! Today we understand that taking care of our body also means taking care of our soul. Below are a few economical and efficient home recipes.

Exfoliation

◎ Take ½ cup of coarse salt and a small bowl of rosemary oil, as a toning solution.
◎ Immerse your exfoliating tool in the rosemary, then in the salt and massage your body in circular motions with particular attention to your articulations (knees, elbows . . .)
◎ Rinse with lukewarm water. Apply a hydrating solution.

Chocolate hydrating solution

◎ Pleasant and suitable for any skin type!
◎ Mix 2 tablespoons of unsweetened cacao with 1 tablespoon of crème fraîche and 1 teaspoon of vegetable oil (your choice).
◎ Leave on the skin for 20 to 30 minutes. Rinse with lukewarm water.

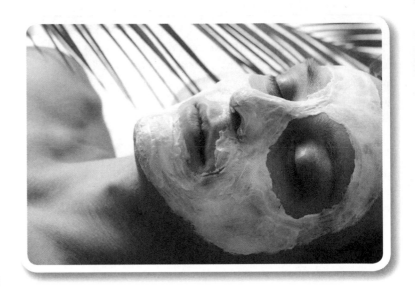

De-stressing citrus bath

◎ Take ¼ cup of lemon zest, ¼ cup of orange zest, 1 tablespoon of dried parsley, and 1 tablespoon of dried comfrey.
◎ Put all the ingredients in your bathtub; run a lukewarm bath and soak for 20 minutes in this balmy citrus bath.

Eye appeasing treatment

◎ Cornflower hydrolat is perfect to relax your eyes strained by hours spent in front of a screen.
◎ Put a few drops on two cotton rounds and apply on your closed eyes.
◎ Lie down for 15 minutes. Experience a deep relaxation.

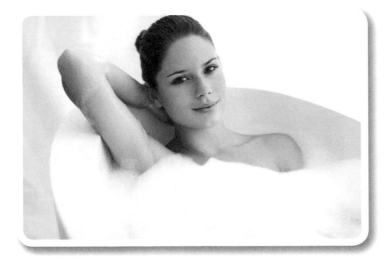

My anti-stress moment

"Drowning." "Losing it." These expressions take their full meaning when stress overwhelms us. Regular walks, even slow and short, allow our body to perform a number of indispensable nervous adjustments.

Below are several examples of de-stress walks. The regularity of the practice is what counts! During the first few minutes, your system coordinates body and breath rhythms. At the beginning, listen to your body: no need to start briskly when you already are anxious or tired. This is the major mistake runners make!

Walk to lower the dominant mental alert

1. Start walking slowly. When you feel your blood circulating properly, you are revved up and ready to increase your rhythm.

2. Consciously concentrate on an object far in front of you: a tree, a field, a street light, a block of houses. At the same time, let your thoughts wander. As soon as your mind starts daydreaming, go back to your objective.

3. Walk for at least ten minutes. Then, rub your thigh muscles.

Walk to refocus

A variant of the first walk, it alternates forward and backward walks. Look down going forward, up going backwards. This will balance your brain. Note that walking backwards works the anterior thigh muscles (like stairs do!).

Walk to relax

Choose a particular place for its natural beauty or peacefulness. Walk and let your eyes wander without analyzing or consciously concentrating. Soak in the atmosphere. Emotions should flow freely.

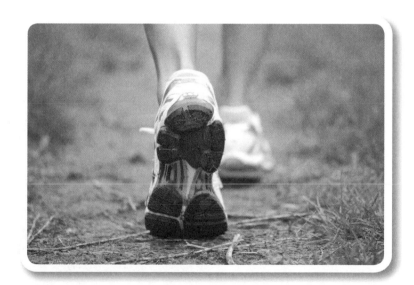

WALKING REGULATES ANXIETY.

My art therapy moment

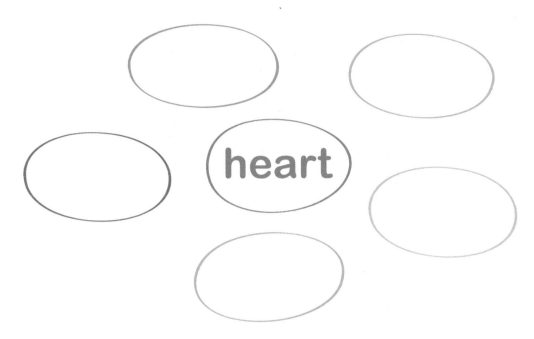

✏️ Express your feelings

◎ When reviewing your life, it is vital to express your feelings. It will prevent you from hitting a brick wall or taking immature decisions driven by emergency or emotions. At the center of this Mind Map, write the word "heart." Use the speech bubbles surrounding it to write the first names of people around you. Trace lines between each bubble and the central heart bubble, then indicate on each line the possible evolution of the relationship between people that are connected. You can add bubbles if necessary.

◎ In a few words, write what amount of personal change would be necessary for these relationships to become constructive:

. . . .
. . . .
. . . .
. . . .
. . . .
. . . .
. . . .
. . . .
. . . .
. . . .
. . . .
. . . .

Meditate on this sentence:

Being alive doesn't suffice. One has to live in the moment, with the knowledge of being at the center of a miracle, and in contact, in harmony with it.

René Barjavel

Health Tip
To assuage your emotions, slowly massage the center of your palms for a few minutes.

My path to well-being

In keeping with the theme of walks, you are going to progressively construct a more intense relationship with your deep self. American Indians call this a "vision walk." This type of internal questioning brings responses that might not make sense right away, as if you needed to mature into them.

◎ First, question yourself on a topic you would like to act upon. For example: what should I do to mend my relationship with (a person close to you)?

◎ Walk slowly, then accelerate progressively; think about this person, about an episode during which the relationship didn't go well. Try to think about it without adding any cumbersome thought.

◎ Wrap the scene with positive emotions; shine a respectful light on it, even if it was violent. You are trying to get some perspective on the event without engulfing yourself in heavy feelings.

◎ Even if it is difficult, think positively; identify the reflections and reactions these moments brought on. Let the scene dissipate.

◎ Now visualize this person out of context: smiling, extending a hand to you. With your soul and your heart, make peace with the person.

◎ Formulate your question, for example: how is the situation between this person and me going to evolve? Mentally formulate it while intently concentrating.

◎ Walk a little longer, letting what is around you sink in. You might have a direct sign, an animal coming towards you, a ray of sun cutting through a gray sky.

◎ Let it go, a dream will perhaps bring a clear response to your question.

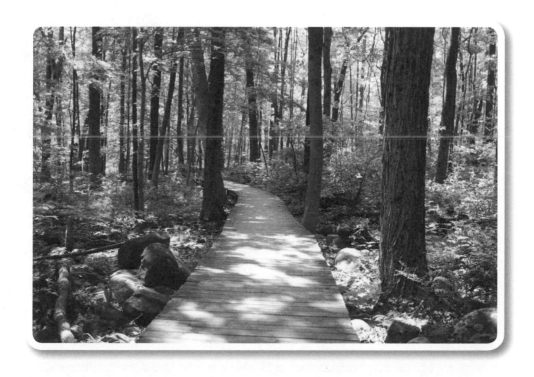

My cocooning space

Soups provide plenty of energy while being light to digest. Perfect for the whole family!

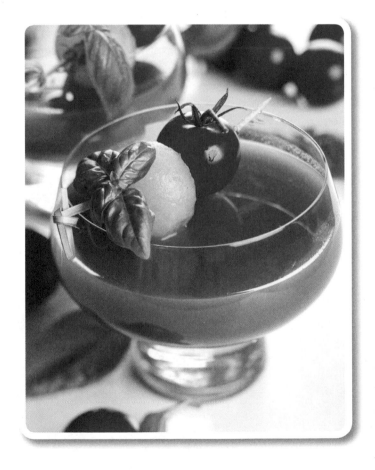

Below are a few tasty and vitamin-rich recipes. Think about including your children in the preparation. Knowledge transmission is important.

Cold avocado soup

◎ Purée 4 avocados with 2 peeled yellow onions.
◎ Add the juice of 1 lemon, 8 ounces of liquid cream, 5 ounces of plain yogurt, 5 ounces of unsweetened milk, and 5 ounces of regular whole milk in a food processor.
◎ Mix to obtain a homogenous smooth potage. Add salt and pepper. Chill for at least 30 minutes before serving.

Cold cucumber soup

◎ Cut both ends of 1 cucumber, then cut it in four pieces to take the seeds out. Chop into very small pieces.
◎ Transfer to a bowl. Add 40 ounces of Bulgarian or Greek yogurt, 1 pressed garlic clove, a few leaves of washed fresh mint, and the chopped cucumber.
◎ Add salt and pepper. Chill for 1 hour. Add lemon before serving.

Cold tomato soup

◎ Purée 4 peeled tomatoes with 1 yellow onion, 1 garlic clove, the juice of 1 lemon, 30 ounces of olive oil, 3 basil leaves, salt, and pepper in a blender.
◎ Chill for 1 hour before serving.

Cold Russian soup

◎ Peel and cut ½ pound of red beets.
◎ Mince 1 fresh fennel bulb, wash and mince ½ cucumber, and peel and grate 1 black radish.
◎ Put all the ingredients in a pot with 1.5 liters of water. Cover and let simmer for 2 hours.
◎ Once cooked, add the juice of 1 lemon, 5 ounces of crème fraîche and purée in a blender. Add freshly cut chives before serving.

My anti-stress moment

On the spot de-stressing is the occasion to get rid of tensions or anxiety. Below are a few techniques you can discreetly use in often stressful situations (Sales meetings, dentist appointments, etc.).

Sitting on the edge of a seat

◎ Palms around your knees, inhale while squeezing your knees in and slightly bending your torso forward.
◎ Exhale while letting go of your knees and coming back to your initial position. Try to do this as slowly as possible.
◎ Inhale while pushing your knees down and planting the arch of your feet on the ground; then exhale and relax.
◎ Repeat both exercises at least three times.

With pen and paper

◎ From a dot in the center of a sheet of paper, scribble lines ending at the top of the sheet. At the same time, think about getting rid of your stress.
◎ Then, still starting from that central point, scribble lines going downward, imagining that you only attract positive thoughts.

Express massage

◎ Discretely, tug at the edge of both your ear lobes for a while. Fold your ear lobes in gently.
◎ Relax all your face muscles. Massage your temples with your index and rub either side of your nose bridge.

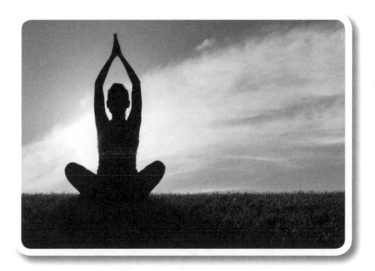

CUT STRESS AT THE ROOT!

My art therapy moment

My important people

◎ Be it regret or frustrating longing, who would you like to see again, or welcome in your life? Start by adding the silhouette of a person (even schematic) on the path, or write a name. If you want to give this encounter a more personal touch, color the scenery as well.

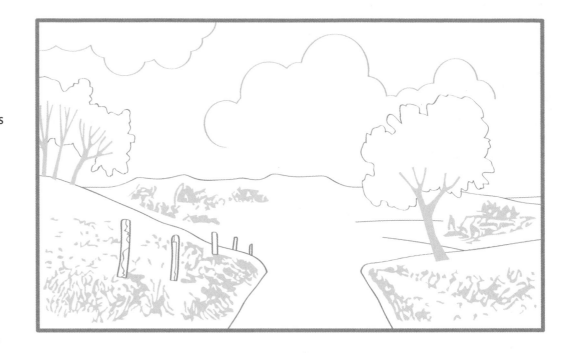

◎ In a few words, write what you would like to share with this person:

. . . .
. . . .
. . . .
. . . .
. . . .
. . . .
. . . .
. . . .
. . . .
. . . .
. . . .
. . . .
. . . .

Meditate on this sentence:

One caress and we emerge from infancy. One word of love and we are born.

Paul Éluard

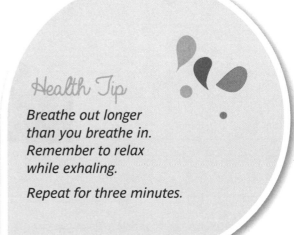

Health Tip

Breathe out longer than you breathe in. Remember to relax while exhaling.

Repeat for three minutes.

My path to well-being

Water is an essential element for everybody's well-being. Below is a path you can adapt to your own situation.

Shower

◎ Using your showerhead massage function (if it has one), massage your head. Close your eyes while mentally feeling the water bring you peace.

◎ Insist on your back muscles and on your nape. Consciously relax while you exhale.

◎ Facing the shower, massage your torso. Then, if you can detach the showerhead, massage from your plexus down to your stomach and work on your intestines. Spend time on each of your thighs and shins.

◎ Finally, with your showerhead at maximum strength, massage your bent knees, one at a time, then your soles.

◎ Finish with a vertical massage from head to toe. Repeat several times.

Bath

◎ Use relaxing essential oils like marjoram, chamomile, and lavender in a lukewarm bath. If at all possible, use organic essential oils.

Pool

◎ Do laps (ideal for the back) or practice slow and controlled movements in the shallow end. Water resistance works wonders on the joints.

Listening

◎ Back straight, sit and meditate listening to the sound of water, either on the bank of a stream or river, on a beach, or simply listening to music. When a thought comes to your mind, re-focus your attention on the sound of the water.

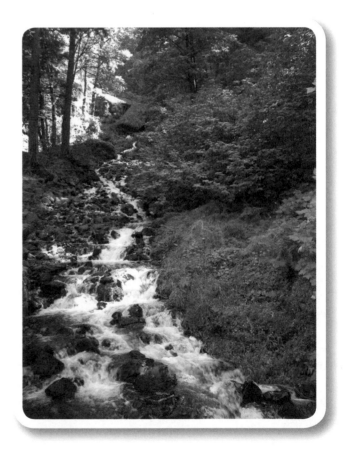

DRINK MINERAL OR FLAT WATER. AVOID CARBONATED WATER, IF POSSIBLE.

My cocooning space

Essential oil diffusers are becoming more and more common in offices and homes. They can appease, energize, induce sleep, or simply add a fresh note to your environment. Below are a few olfactory ideas.

 Mix equal parts of . . .

◎ To dissipate an aggressive mental mood: ravintsara, marjoram, and mandarin.

◎ For agitated children (3 years and older): same as above plus rosemary and chamomile.

◎ For anxiety: geranium, lavender, and sandalwood.

◎ For congested lungs: myrtle, palmarosa, rosemary, and ravintsara.

◎ To foster concentration: basil, mint, and Scotch pine.

◎ For a depressive spell: ylang-ylang, small grain bigarade, and ravintsara.

◎ For physical fatigue: black spruce, peppermint, and Scotch pine.

◎ For sore throat: tea tree, lemon, mint, and thyme.

◎ For headaches: sandalwood, tea tree, and thyme.

◎ For sinus infections: pine tree, eucalyptus, and peppery mint.

◎ For difficulty falling asleep: ravintsara, myrtle, and lemon verbena.

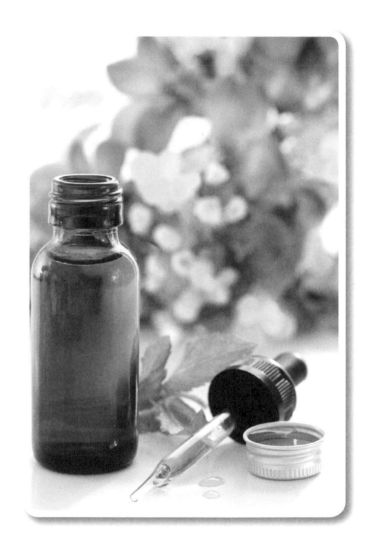

My anti-stress moment

A twenty-minute relaxation session equals two hours of sleep.

Lying down, inhale through your nose and inflate your stomach while concentrating on the part of your body that needs to relax. Then, inhale through your mouth (or nose) adding the intention to totally relax the targeted spot.

You can associate images to visualizing the part of your body, like a calm lake, a serene blue sky, a peaceful scene. Motivate yourself with positive sentences: "I feel good," "I am open to the world," "I am receptive."

1. Start by concentrating on each element of your face: your lids, your eyebrows, your forefront, all your scalp, the sides of your nose, your cheekbones, your cheeks, the ear area, the chin. Insist on unlocking your jaws and lips. Then on to your shoulders, arms, elbows, forearms, wrists, and hands.

2. Go on to your nape and backbone. Progressively go down to your hips and relax all the muscles on either side of the backbone, making sure to relax the lumbar area.

3. Continue with the chest, the sides, your waist, and the abdominal belt.

4. Also relax the hips, buttock, perineum, thighs, knees, shins, ankles, and feet, all the way to your toes.

5. Finish by imagining the energy harmoniously spreading and going back up your head. After stretching your hands and feet, open your eyes, or go to sleep . . .

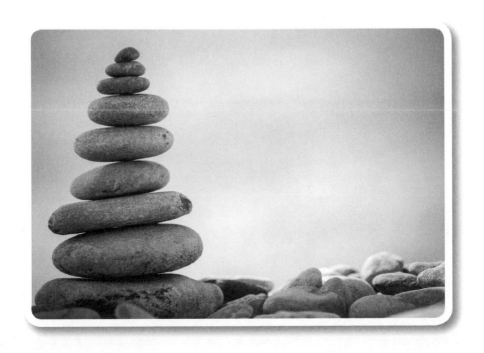

My art therapy moment

Know how to take root

◎ Connecting to your roots evokes gathering one's strength from one's parcel of land, your own inner scenery. Center yourself on your present needs. First, color the roots and add words referring to the foundation of your life. Then, the branches and the leaves, coloring and writing what you are hoping for.

◎ In a few words, describe how you could make this tree grow even more:

....

....

....

....

....

....

....

....

....

....

....

....

....

....

....

....

....

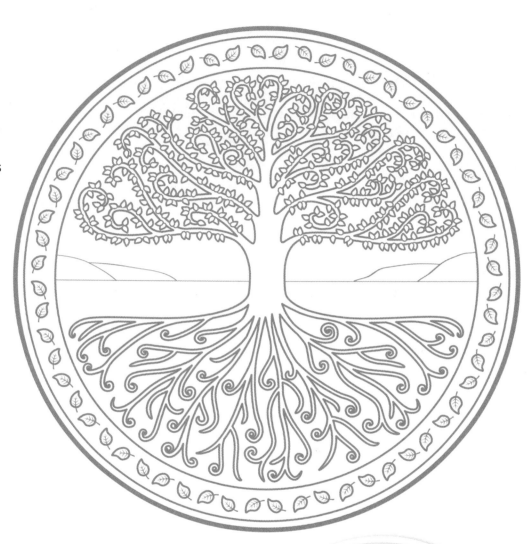

Meditate on this sentence:

What death is to a caterpillar, a butterfly calls rebirth.

Violette Lebon

Health Tip

To find deep peace, massage your stomach clockwise with your palms while breathing slowly.

74

My path to well-being

Let's associate a few simple yoga poses to the warm up and stretching exercises you have already mastered. Always make sure your practice is progressive and breathe through the effort. Results are not impacted by how long you hold the pose. Be present, be in the "here and now" and listen to your body. Below is a basic course.

1. Standing up, legs apart, inhale with your arms extended. Exhale while bending your torso forward. Concentrate on relaxing your whole back.

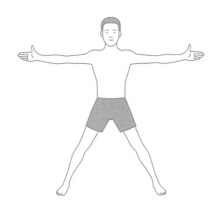

2. Turn your head to the right, lifting your right arm toward the ceiling. With your left arm, reach toward or touch your left ankle. Come back to your original position and switch sides. Repeat two more times on either side.

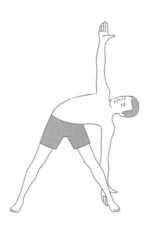

3. Fix your eyes on a point on the ground. Your arms slightly away from your body, bring your right foot onto your left thigh or calf.

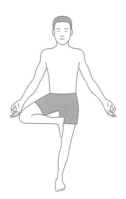

4. Keep the pose for a few minutes, calmly breathing in and out. Then join your palms on your plexus.

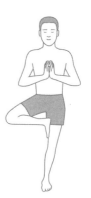

5. Breathe in and out while keeping the pause, then bring your hands on top of your head. Feel your entire body, the tensions and relaxations.

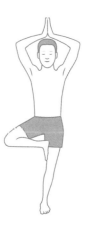

Repeat twice, rest, and drink some water.

My cocooning space

Herbal teas are your health's best friends. Here are a few simple but useful choices. We suggest you buy only the quantity you need from an herbalist so as to dispense with the arduous process of preserving the herbs at home.

Angst

◎ Avoid stimulants like alcohol or coffee; practice relaxation and eat read meat in moderation.
◎ Three cups a day of: 1.4 ounces of eschscholtzia leaves, 2.8 ounces of passionflower, 1.4 ounces of red poppy petals, and 2.8 ounces of orange tree leaves. Steep 0.7 ounces of this mix in 1 liter of boiling water for 10 minutes.

Bronchitis

◎ Rest and light food are in order.
◎ Four cups a day of: 2.8 ounces of eucalyptus leaves, 0.9 ounces of white marrube (horehound) leaves, 2.6 ounces of Scotch pine blooms, and 1.7 ounces of erysimum. Steep 0.7 ounces of this mix in 1 liter of boiling water for 10 minutes.

Conjunctivitis

◎ Avoid sun or closed spaces.
◎ For an eye bath, mix 2.8 ounces of cornflower, 3.5 ounces of chamomile flowers, and 1.05 ounces of plantain leaves. Steep 1.7 ounces of this mix in 1 liter of boiling water for 10 minutes.
◎ Let the infusion cool. Put a few drops on cotton rounds. Apply on your eyelids several times a day.

Insomnia

◎ Practice relaxation and sophrology.
◎ Mix 1.7 ounces each of hawthorn flower clusters, passionflower, orange, and linden. Steep 0.7 ounces of this mix in 1 liter of boiling water for 10 minutes. Drink 1 cup before going to bed.

Heart palpitations

◎ Practice a physical activity regularly and try to keep a healthy weight.
◎ Mix 1.7 ounces each of hawthorn, passionflower, red poppy, and verbena odorosa. Steep 0.7 ounces of this mix in 1 liter of boiling water for 10 minutes. Drink 3 cups a day.

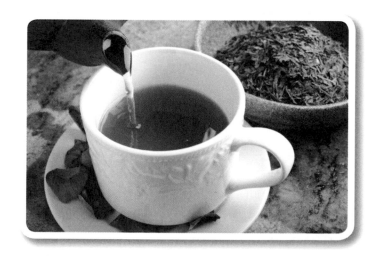

REGULAR SEASONAL HERBAL TEA BREAKS ARE A TREAT.

My anti-stress moment

Should you ask the right questions or trust a confident *laissez-faire*? Stress accumulates because certain events are not considered or solved, making it necessary to keep a journal of your needs, or formal review. This is not monitoring. It is deserved self-respect!

1. Invest in an attractive notebook (not mourning black or blood red). Dedicate a pen to those personal moments.

2. On the left page, enter the signs of stress you can identify: nervousness, irritability, loss of appetite, increased food intake, etc. Then, list your stresses and rank them, "one" being the lowest.

3. On the right page, indicate each stress trigger: difficult hierarchical relationships, children going through aggressive stages, etc.

4. Trace lines between the two pages for each possible interaction. You very probably will conclude that one event can generate several stresses. Moreover, secondary stress sources accumulate and amplify the primary sources. You might even discover that one stress you consider less important triggers many others much more difficult to manage!

5. Write simple solutions you should implement to improve the situation. Perform your formal review every fifteen days. With time, priorities will evolve and stress will become more manageable.

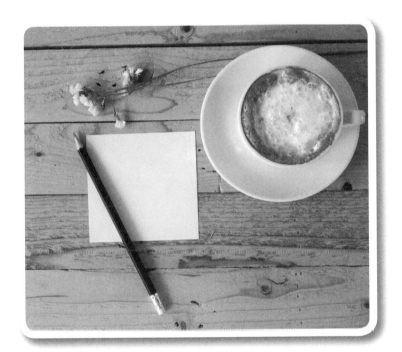

IDENTIFYING ITS SOURCES DIFFUSES YOUR STRESS.

My art therapy moment

Open your heart

◎ Use this time to diffuse your stress with light and harmonious colors. The louder your heart talks, the less your stress screams!

Meditate on this sentence:

The heart never lies.

Reis Mirdita

◎ In a few words, describe what an affair of the heart is for you:

. . . .
. . . .
. . . .
. . . .
. . . .
. . . .
. . . .
. . . .
. . . .
. . . .
. . . .
. . . .

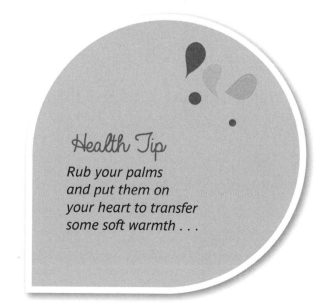

Health Tip

Rub your palms and put them on your heart to transfer some soft warmth . . .

My path to well-being

For your second yoga experience, simply repeat last week's warm-up. Slowly follow the pleasant path below. The "weighing scale" pose brings mental balance. The important point is to alternate concentration and relaxation (a Westerner's dream!)

1. Start on the floor, your buttocks on your heels, hands on your thighs. Calmly breathe while concentrating on a point in front of you. Then put your palms together and bring them up above your head while inhaling. Move your buttocks towards your right heel and slowly curve your body to the left, turning your head to the right.

3. Take a two-minute pause. Sit up on the floor, feet planted on your mat. Bend your right leg parallel to the floor, right foot to your left buttock. Place your left palm on your side for support. Slowly bring your left foot over your right knee. Grab your left ankle with your right hand. While breathing in, slowly turn your head to the left; invest time in relaxing the right side of your body. Repeat the exercise three times on either side.

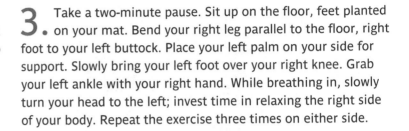

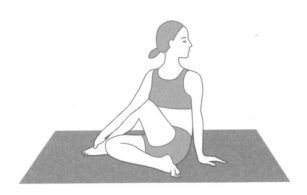

2. Feeling your spine stretch, round your arms and breathe out. Come back to your original position and repeat twice on the same side. Switch sides and repeat three times. Pay attention to your stomach every time you exhale.

4. Sitting up, bring your soles together, knees as far down as you can. Pass your hands through your bended legs and bring them on your feet. Slowly, exhale while your body goes forward. Rest while relaxing your back.

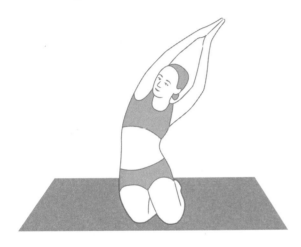

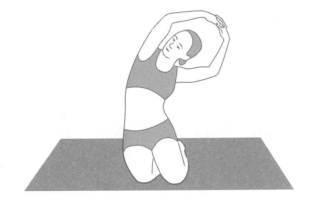

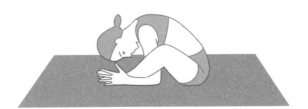

My cocooning space

 Cocooning also means reclaiming your taste buds by using what Mother Nature offers us. Below are a few simple and affordable recipes to share with friends or family.

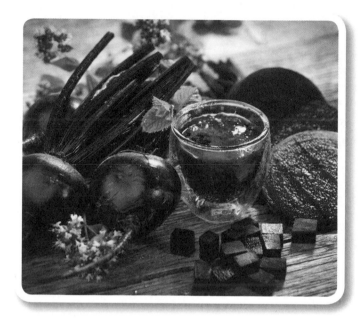

Garlic Bouillon

You need: 2 cloves of garlic per person, a few almonds, and walnuts.

◎ Cook all the ingredients in 1 liter of water for 20 minutes at low heat.

◎ Filter the bouillon and serve it in a bowl, accompanied by a slice of bread on which you place garlic, walnuts, and almonds. Excellent for hypertension!

Red Beet Juice

You need: 1 pound of raw beets.

◎ Cut the beets in thin slices, put them in a bowl, and cover with water. Let sit overnight. In the morning, purée in a blender. One glass is ideal for anemia or for a vitamin boost.

Apricot Syrup

You need: 2 pounds of sugar for 2 pounds of apricots.

◎ Slowly cook the ingredients for 15 minutes. Let cool, filter, and put in a bottle.

◎ Some syrup in a glass of ice-cold water makes for a refreshing drink!

Carrot Syrup

You need: 2 pounds of carrots, 1 liter of water, and ½ pound of sugar.

◎ Wash and peel the carrots.

◎ Add sugar and carrots to 1 liter of boiling water. Cook 2 hours on low heat.

◎ Allow to cool, filter, and reserve in a bottle. Serve with a few drops of lemon juice. Yum!

Acacia Flower Lemonade

You need: 1 big handful of acacia flowers, 1 lemon, and 2 teaspoons of powdered sugar.

◎ In the morning put the acacia flowers in a 1-liter bottle. Fill with water, add 2 slices of lemon, and leave in the sun all day.

◎ At the end of the day, add the sugar. Place the bottle in a cool place. It is ready to drink in the morning. Delicious thirst quencher!

Cherry Stems Infusion

You need: 1.8 ounces cherry stems.

◎ Drop the cherry stems in 1 liter of boiling water. Steep 10 minutes. Very efficient to calm rheumatisms and prevent the flu!

My anti-stress moment

Here is an anti-stress toolbox, which is useful to dispel specific daily stresses!

◎ General muscular tension: gently tug on your ear lobes. Continue delicately rolling the cartilaginous part of your outer ear toward the inside. Using your index finger, massage each side of your jaw by pushing it and letting go. Preventively, repeat five minutes every two hours.

◎ Sudden anxiety and panic attack: bend your arms over your chest, your hands are back to back with your fingers clinched as much as you can. Cross your legs and keep your tongue pushed on your palate. Breathe regularly, until your anxiety subsides.

◎ Visual fatigue: warm up your palms by rubbing them together. Cover your eyes with your warm hands for a while, imagining that your palms are absorbing the stress and appeasing your brain.

◎ General tiredness: massage the meaty part of your thumb close to your wrist. Switch hands.

◎ Emotional tensions: using your two index fingers, find the natural hollow points on the line between your breasts and gently massage them to restore emotional peace.

◎ Stomach tensions: with your left index finger, find the middle point between your right thumb and your index finger. If painful, your stomach is upset! Switch sides.

◎ Mental tension: lift your hair strand by strand to massage the entirety of your scalp. Using your ten fingers, massage your whole scalp as if shampooing.

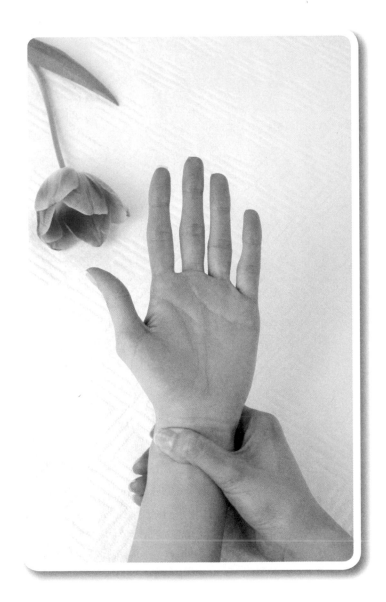

SPECIFIC STRESSES CALL FOR TARGETED ACTIONS.

My art therapy moment

 Emotional evaluation

◎ Let the sun shine and warm up your heart. Color its rays, using happy colors for the earth, a symbolic representation of yourself.

◎ In a few words, define what you need to facilitate your personal progression:

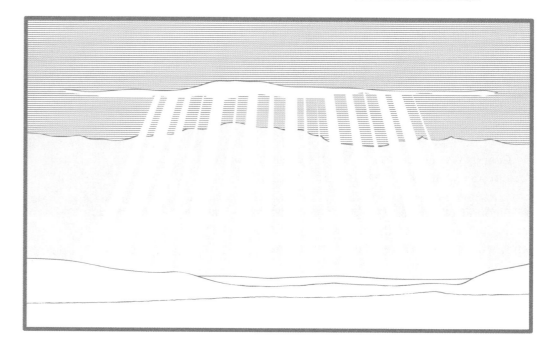

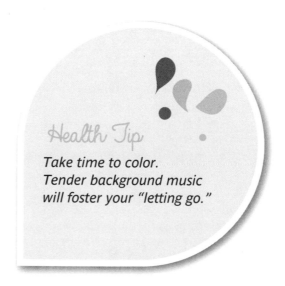

Health Tip

Take time to color. Tender background music will foster your "letting go."

My path to well-being

This is your third yoga session. Adapt it to your level, it is not a competition!

1. After warming up, sit up on your mat, legs extended, feet at a forty-five degree angle. Inhale while lifting both arms. Bring your palms together.

3. Lie on your stomach, elbows, arms, and palms on the mat. Inhale while lifting your head and slowly extending your arms to lift your torso, slightly tilting your head back. Your palms stabilize the pose. Exhale and concentrate on your chest opening fully and your back relaxing. Slowly come back to your original position. Repeat three times or more.

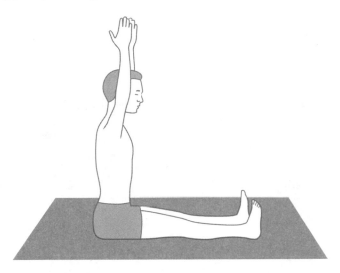

2. Stay in apnea for a short moment. Exhale while bending your torso towards your feet. If available to you, touch your toes with your hands.

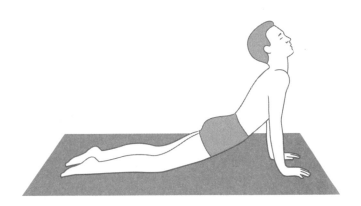

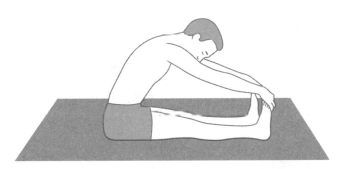

BODY FLEXIBILITY PREVENTS MUSCULAR TENSIONS.

My cocooning space

Every single crystal has its specific transparency and structure. Crystals are used in telecommunication and computer chips because they are said to concentrate energy. Program a crystal to enhance your well-being.

Your security crystal

◎   In a mineral rock store, buy the hardest crystal available, four inches maximum. Make sure no edge is broken. Crystals capture all frequencies, so bury yours or put it in a container filled with clean water overnight. Then put it in the sun, even if dim, from morning to 3PM.

◎   Take your crystal in your hand. Imagine that you are delicately opening its seven petals as if it were a flower. By establishing an intimate relationship with this transparent crystal you are opening the energetic heart of the crystal, making it receptive. First, concentrate on what would be most useful to you every day. For example: "When I need energy, I think about you. You send me strength wherever I am." Now concentrate on the crystal and see yourself programming that thought into the crystal.

◎   Mentally close back each petal one by one. Amplify its energy by placing the crystal on your heart, feel that you are giving it some of your personal energy, too. Every day get in touch with your crystal, reformulate your creative thought: "When I need energy, I think about you, you send me your strength no matter where I am." Feel your energy increase. You can also use a crystal for your child. Choose a sentence like: "With you, I am not afraid during the night." You can also place the crystal under your child's pillow!

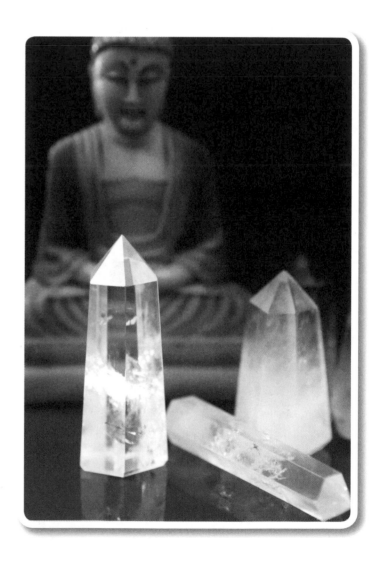

Local Exchanges

Making the general public aware of local exchanges is a great way to contribute. Today, a large number of associations and volunteers coordinate their energies to develop new, durable local exchanges.

Currently, anybody can establish a list of addresses and references that is easily disseminated either on a dedicated site or during local events. Municipalities can be contacted directly.

Depending on what is available in your area, you will need to start from scratch or enrich what is already available.

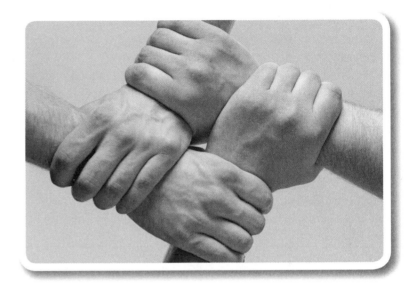

Local Exchange Trading System (LETS)

A Local Exchange Trading System (LETS) is a local organization that allows members to participate in an exchange of goods, services, and know-hows with others in the group, without the use of money.

Some LETS use "exchange sheets" (or "wealth sheets") on which participants note with whom they exchange and how many units have to be credited or debited (depending on time spent or type of exchange).

Others use three-flap coupons (two for the participants of the exchange, one for the LETS "accountant")

Local Currencies

The objective of a local currency is to reinforce the notion of community participation in a defined area. For example, *l'Occitan* (the local money in Pézenas, France) is a loyalty tool for all the participants, since it only can be expended within the precise confines of the community.

It creates a monetary mass—a captive buying power necessarily reinvested locally—that will not be lost in the arcane meanders of obscure financial investments. It is not speculative since it doesn't produce interest and has a one-year lifespan.

START A COMMUNITY SYSTEM TO SIMPLIFY MEMBERS' LIVES.

Group Creativity

Nowadays, children gladly engage in electronic activities. Why not surf the Internet to access the information used in a communal fresco?

◎ The idea is to create a fresco, a "wall" of first names.

◎ Start by choosing a "referring" family to give a presentation of the project at the local school, municipality, etc.

◎ You need a temporary surface, several municipal boards or school blackboards covered with white sheets of paper, a wall, etc., on which to exhibit the first name fresco (obtain official permission). It will be unveiled during a community event, i.e. on the last day of school or during a local fair.

◎ **First phase:** create a box in which participants can contribute a first name. Use either a physical box with a drop slot, pen and paper, or a virtual box created on a community site.

◎ **Second phase:** the project leader catalogs the first names and makes the list available to the participating teachers. Each child adds a word by each first name: sun, nice, blue . . . Let the children be creative.

◎ **Third phase:** children participating in transcribing first names and associated words are chosen by consensus. They use color crayons to realize the fresco.

◎ **The finished fresco** will be accessible to all—children and parents. It will be an occasion, notably for the adults, to become aware (and surprised at times!) of the role children attribute to first names. It will generate interesting discussions on the cultural aspect of first names and illustrate the community's cultural diversity.

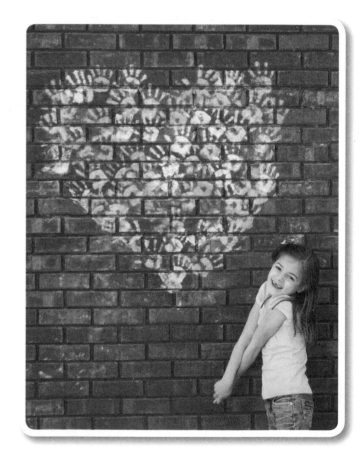

Art therapy collective

Mind Mapping® is an activity that establishes a "map" of information available on one subject in order to start a reflection on the topic. Below is a plan you can use for the topic of your choice. The objective here is to bring family, friends, or neighbors together for this Mind Mapping session.

◎ Place the topic in the center of the blackboard. For example: Travel.

◎ First, each participant uses one of the spaces left open to write, color, or glue an image, to express thoughts about travel, keeping in mind that each participant should leave space for the others. If need be, create a second board for participants to unpack their ideas.

◎ Then, every one returns to the Mind Map and links ideas that seem common or complementary.

◎ Finally, all the participants discuss the topic.

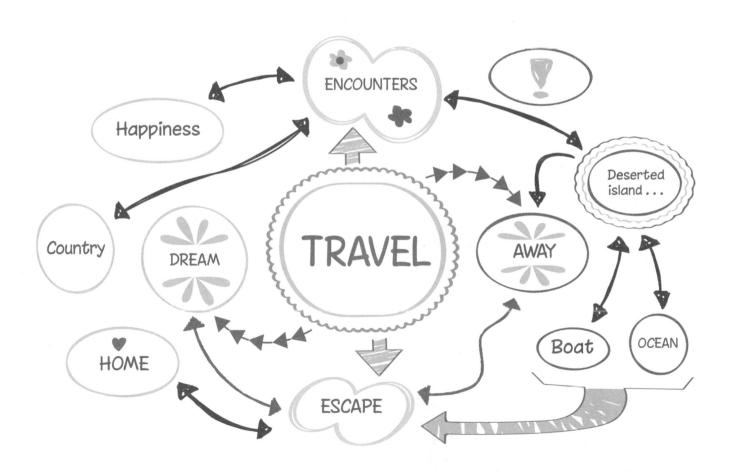

My anti-stress moment

Repeating some methods and putting them to the test also teaches us to de-stress. Bring your smile, your personal interests, and the words that matter to you as you engage in your well-being process. Characterize this newfound relaxation by a generic theme. Light is the synthetic element of our relaxation. White at first, it can become blue if more peaceful to you, green for more oxygen or for healing. . . . Practice at least once a week to benefit from its positive impact.

1. Lie down and close your eyes. Breathe in and out deeply. When inhaling, let the air into your stomach first, then into your chest. Repeat three times.

2. Contract all the muscles of your body for a few seconds. Release all of them.

3. Imagine a soft white light entering your body through your toes. Feel its effect without becoming too tense, trying to visualize the light. Simply direct your attention to your wish to relax.

4. Keep in mind that this light stands for calm, relaxation, peace, and quiet, and that your whole body profits from it, quietly and softly.

5. Slowly, see the white light go along your legs. Feel that it frees your feet, your shins, your knees, your thighs. The light is brighter and brighter and goes up your stomach, your chest. Then it flows into your arms and your hands. Finally, the bright light flows into your head, relaxing each muscle of your face. As if a magic broom appeared, feel the light sweeping you, from your feet to your head. Experience harmony.

6. Progressively, add the words you need: soft light, cool or warm light, energizing or peaceful . . .

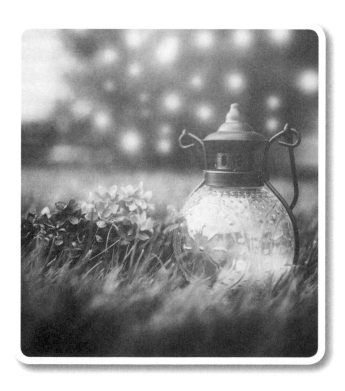

My art therapy moment

✏️ Representing light

◎ This aurora borealis symbolically represents all the light you need to regenerate yourself. Choose its colors according to your own energy needs.

◎ In a few words, write what the word "light" represents for you:

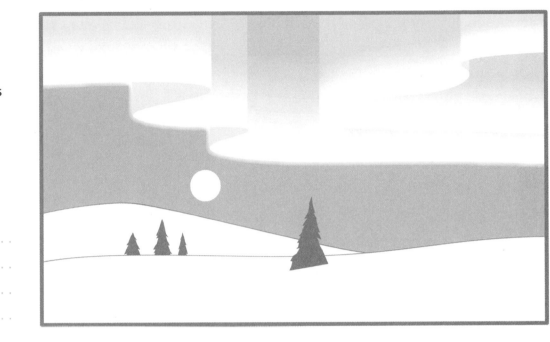

Meditate on this sentence:

Light is not missing in our gaze; our gaze is missing the light.

Gustave Thibon

Health Tip

To soothe your visual system, place a green cloth in front of your eyes and intently look at it for a few minutes without thinking about anything. Repeat regularly.

My path to well-being

When it comes to relaxing, Cat and Cow poses are simple and extremely efficient. Follow the drawings below. Associate the proper breathing to each pose. Progressively and at your own pace, add more poses.

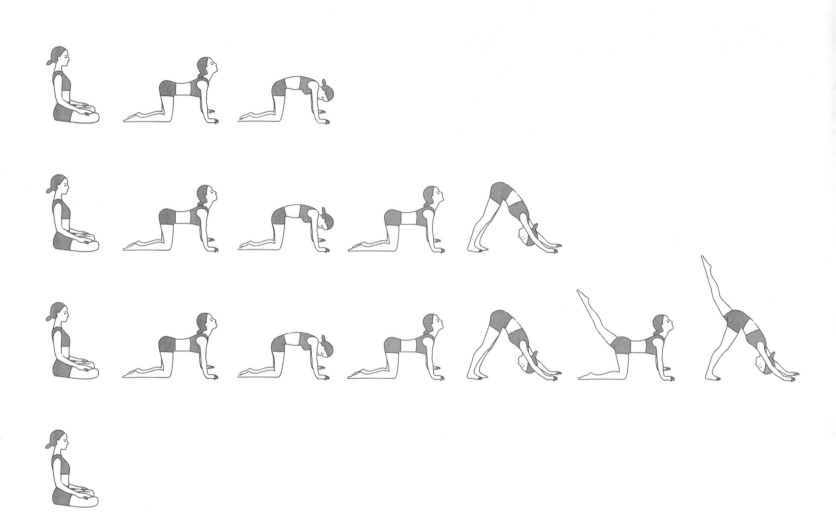

My cocooning space

A concrete and original way to keep in touch with nature and its four seasons—even in an urban setting—is to create a small-container vegetable garden on a balcony, or an herb pot garden on a windowsill. Here is how to choose:

◎ Choose your plants according to their mature size.

◎ Observe the sun exposure of your window. Fruits need lots of sun, while vegetables prefer some shade.

◎ Plan your access to water. You might have to attach a hose to your kitchen faucet.

◎ Make sure your plants will be attended to (watering, cleaning, etc.)

◎ Inquire to know whether your balcony has a structural weight limit. Does your building regulate the usage of balconies? Inquire with management. Check municipal ordinances.

◎ Examples of easy-to-grow plants: eggplants, beets, carrots, cauliflower, zucchinis, watercress, cherry tomatoes, peppers, radishes, lettuce, basil, thyme, tarragon, and rosemary. Small lemon or orange trees require lots of sun. Something to consider!

◎ Plan where to store your gardening tools. Leave enough space to circulate in your garden.

◎ Look into elevated planters or pots on wheels. They will spare your back and allow you to move your plants around. Convenient!

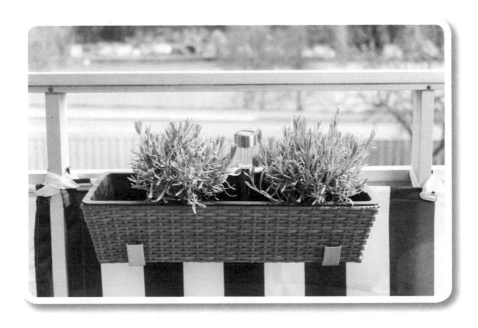

My anti-stress moment

Autosuggestion is a simple way to get a grip on your life by using a conscious mental plan. Not transforming you into a robot, but rather using a technique to act directly on your mind. Often, the stress is such that your brain is beyond your reach, with the ensuing fatigue and/or nervousness that govern your basic reactions. Thanks to autosuggestion, you will take some distance from your conditioning and negative ideas. To that end, you must find words and sentences that do not oppose your conscious to your unconscious (i.e. words that would be contrary to your beliefs). Progressively, this median voice takes root in your subconscious and dominates your conscious.

1. Start by formulating a short sentence that sums up your objective: "Day to day, I am calmer and more relaxed, I don't let stress get to me."

2. It is easier to program your mind through conscious breathing. It will induce alpha brain waves (very close to sleep), foster deep rooting, and implement thinking processes:

◎ start by inhaling and exhaling deeply four times.
◎ breathe in, counting up to five. Keep air in, counting up to seven. Exhale, counting up to nine. Repeat ten to twelve times.

Note: we are not counting seconds. Adapt your breathing rhythm to your lung capacity. If your feel you are hyperventilating, stop the exercise, relax, and go back to it when you are ready.

3. Once relaxed, repeat tirelessly the affirmation sentence with the desire that it be operational, without the shadow of a doubt. Repeat for twenty-one days.

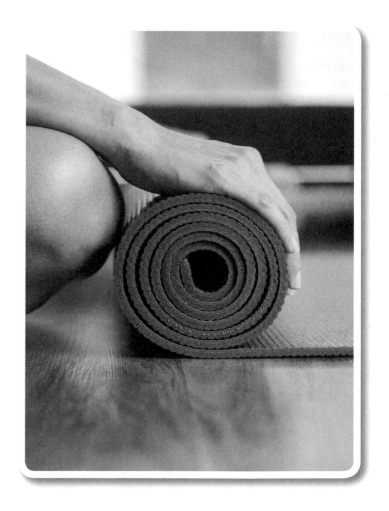

My art therapy moment

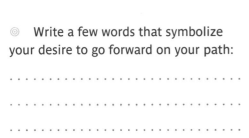 ## Being able to turn the page

◎ Leaving one's past and going forward is based on a desire, a true life-choice. Confirm your commitment by consciously completing the right of this drawing mainly with curves, nourishing the idea of a positive progression towards your future.

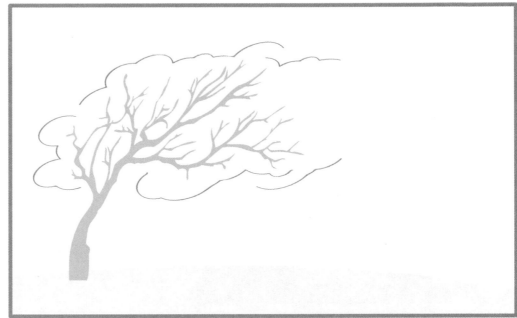

◎ Write a few words that symbolize your desire to go forward on your path:

. . . .
. . . .
. . . .
. . . .
. . . .
. . . .
. . . .
. . . .
. . . .
. . . .
. . . .
. . . .
. . . .
. . . .
. . . .
. . . .

Meditate on this sentence:

The only way to avoid the future is to invent it.

Alan Kay

Health Tip

Take several pauses while coloring to simply relax your ten fingers by clasping your hands together and extending your arms above your head, hands turned over, inhaling, then slowly bringing your arms down on the desk while exhaling.

My path to well-being

Continue your yoga practice with these gentle and relaxing poses.

1. Sit on your heels. Get up on your knees and put your hands behind you while inhaling. Gently bend backwards, feeling the stretch of your whole body. Repeat three times.

3. Sit on your heels. Extend your arms backwards, hands on the floor, palms up. Bend frontward so your forefront touches the floor. Stay in position a few minutes to relax. You can also bring your extended arms to the front, palms on the ground.

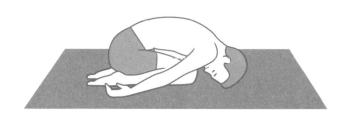

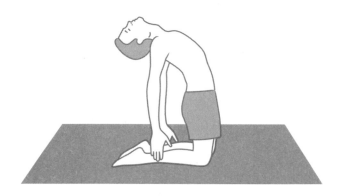

2. Lay on your back. Arms are extended at a forty-five degree angle and palms are on your mat. Turn your head to the right while bringing your folded knees to the left and exhale. Reverse the pose. Repeat the cycle three more times. Feel your back and your lumbar region work.

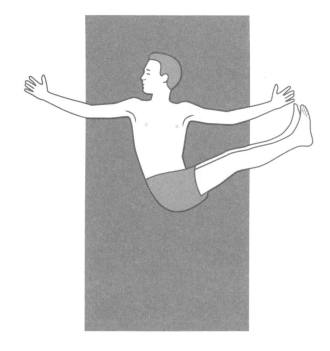

My cocooning space

 Our face contains numerous sensorial receptors. Today, pollution is prevalent, even on top of the highest mountains! Cleaning our face and paying attention to it should be a natural endeavor for women and for men.

Below are a few do-it-yourself skin care treatments suitable for all skin types.

To soothe

◎ In a bowl, whip 2 egg whites, 2 tablespoons of liquid honey, 1 teaspoon of almond oil, and the juice of 1 lemon.
◎ Apply lightly to clean and moist skin, avoiding the eye area.
◎ Keep for 15 minutes and rinse.

To refresh

◎ Slice 1 cucumber without peeling it. Put in a bowl and cover with warm water. Let sit for 1 hour. Drain through a cheesecloth.
◎ Add ½ teaspoon of benzoin tincture. Mix and pour in a glass bottle. Close hermetically.
◎ Keep up to one week in the fridge.

To relax and rejuvenate

◎ Put 1 tablespoon of dry peppermint in a jar. Add ½ cup of hamamelis (witch hazel) water.
◎ Close and let sit for one week, shaking the jar once a day.
◎ Filter and pour the preparation back in the jar, adding ½ cup of rose water and 1 teaspoon of vegetable glycerin.
◎ Shake the jar and apply to the face.

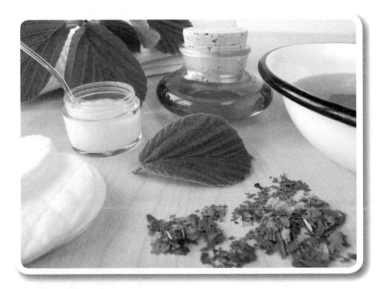

YOUR FACE NEEDS YOUR UNDIVIDED ATTENTION.

My anti-stress moment

In praise of happy trees! The forest is brimming with energy and so are the trees, whether yin or yang. Try this gentle and de-stressing arboreal cuddle.

1. You want to identify a dominant tree, not necessarily the highest one, but the one whose presence speaks to you and makes it stand out from the rest. If its top is flattened, its thick foliage reaching for the earth like an old oak tree, it is because it receives energy from the sky. On the other hand, if it is elegantly soaring (like a poplar), its energy comes from the earth and it is attracted to the sky. Let a tree's energy draw you to it.

2. Once you have identified your tree, lie down and place your bare feet directly on its trunk. Let the gentle energy of the tree flow in your legs and into your body. Take as much time as you need. Let your gaze wander over the bark, the leaves, the foliage. . . .

3. Sit with your back on the tree. Slightly roll right and left so the rough bark massages your back. Kneel facing the tree and put your palms on the bark, close your eyes and feel the tingling and/or the warmth that travel your body. If some of its

roots lie above ground, grab then and mentally "connect" to the telluric energy through those vegetal anchors.

4. Finally, stand up and hug the tree. Then, as previously for your back, roll your torso right and left to massage your bust. Smell the wood, cuddle your friend, your tree.

5. Once relaxed, mentally thank the tree and come back each season to maintain your friendship. Enjoy the atmosphere and the energies of the forest and see it change with each season!

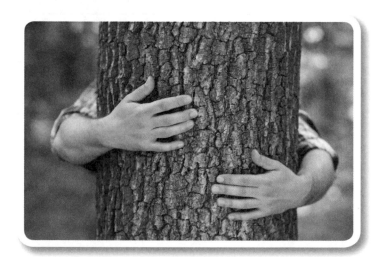

THE TREE'S ENERGY HARMONIZES YOUR AURA.

My art therapy moment

✏️ Gentle force and brute force

◎ Draw the yin, the creative force, with upward coloring pencil strokes. Draw the yang, the brute force, with downward strokes.

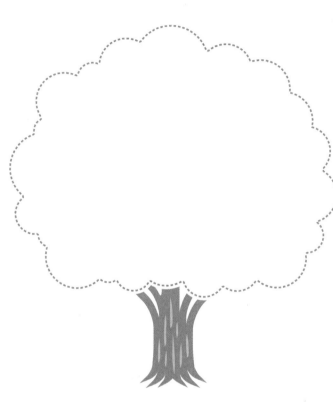

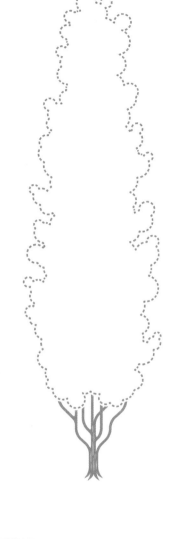

◎ In a few words, describe what you would like to happen when alone in nature:

. . . .

. . . .

. . . .

. . . .

. . . .

. . . .

. . . .

. . . .

. . . .

. . . .

. . . .

. . . .

. . . .

. . . .

. . . .

. . . .

. . . .

. . . .

Meditate on this sentence:

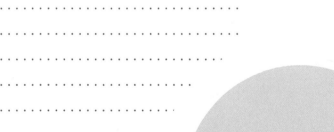

To each their own.

Philibert-Joseph Le Roux

Health Tip

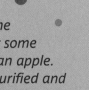

For your walks in the forest, always bring some natural water and an apple. Your body will be purified and recharged by the vitamins and minerals.

My path to well-being

Now that you are familiar with the stretches introduced in the previous yoga sessions, you can start pushing your body a little more, keeping within the limits of what is available to you. Bear in mind that the benefits of the poses depend on your attention to form. You are doing this for your well-being. This salutation to the sun sums up several basic poses.

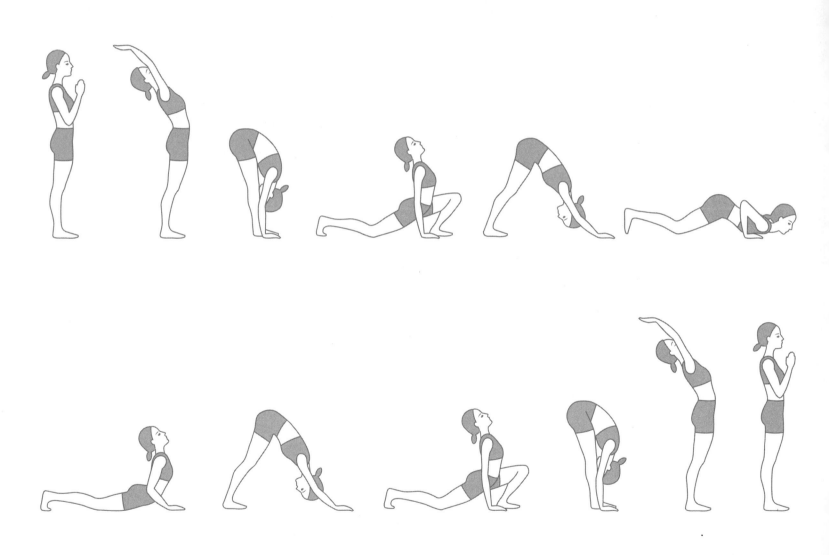

My cocooning space

 Think about using fruit and vegetables for your facial treatments. Try to get the highest quality—no pesticides, organic if possible—particularly when using a zest or an unpeeled fruit.

Cucumber

◎ Rich in water and potassium, cucumber is soothing, hydrating, and re-balances your pH.
◎ It is particularly recommended for the very sensitive skin around the eyes.

Lemon

◎ It is astringent, tonic, and balances your pH. Also efficient for wrinkles and dark spots.
◎ Purifying, smoothing, and lightening.

Grapes

◎ Astringent and rich in minerals, grapes are your skin's best friend.
◎ Tone, hydrate, and lighten.

Red Berries

◎ Detoxifying, they cleanse your blood—therefore your skin—by fostering tissue regeneration.
◎ Their natural pigments promote cell and lesion regeneration.

Carrots

◎ Anti-inflammatory, diuretic, and revitalizing. Use on wrinkles and for skin infections.

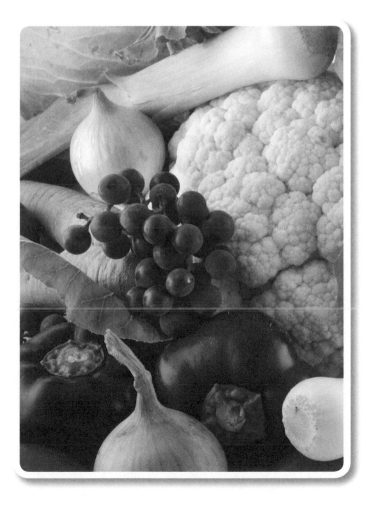

My anti-stress moment

Unpacking words requires reflection and coherence. Here, each word suggests escape, daydreaming, and enjoyment. You are not asked to produce difficult word associations but rather instinctive, almost automatic writing.

◎   Associate a color with each sentence, like a force evoking gentleness and peacefulness. Creativity and imagination will soothe your mind. You can produce a succession of sentences or a structured text, whatever you prefer. Think about breathing gently and preferably write in a calm place.

◎   Proposed words: gentleness, tenderness, calm, appeasement, rejuvenation, "letting go," relaxation, sleep, daydream, wander, exchange, share, moments, instants, clarity, openness, mountain, river, soft waves, soft rain, sun, starry sky, green plants, flowers, colors, garden, laughter, smile, child, fairy, elf, scenery, blue, orange, shrub, fly, pretty, pink stone, ocean, warm wind . . .

◎   Your indispensable words (different from those offered):

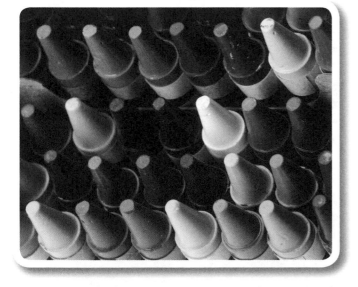

My art therapy moment

✏️ **Reviewing**

◎ How do you feel about your life today? You are in the center of the drawing. Start by adding the color that corresponds best to you, then evolve towards the edges imagining the colors you are bringing with you (happy, pleasant, or unpleasant?)

◎ In a few words, explain the reasons you chose those colors:

. . . .
. . . .
. . . .
. . . .
. . . .
. . . .
. . . .
. . . .
. . . .
. . . .
. . . .
. . . .
. . . .
. . . .
. . . .
. . . .
. . . .
. . . .

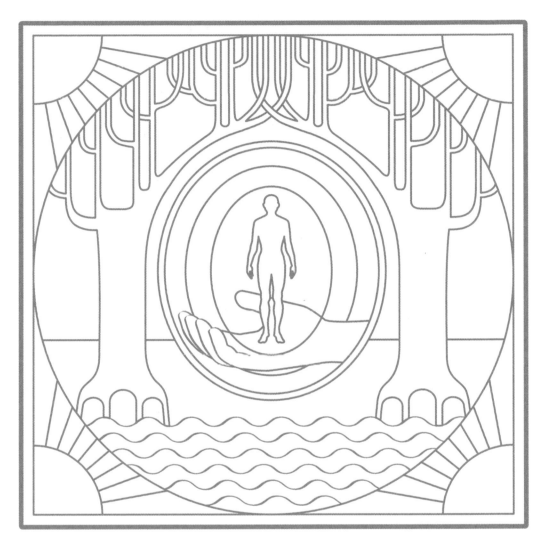

Meditate on this sentence:

Clarity adorns deep thoughts.

Luc de Clapiers,
Marquis de Vauvenargues

Health Tip

Take a few moments to breathe calmly and balance your head by making a 360 degree circle one way, then the other, in order to relax.

My path to well-being

To continue with our posture, this path is particularly appropriate for those who spend most of their day sitting, whether in a vehicle or in front of a computer screen. Be gentle and practice this series once in the morning and once in the afternoon, if possible.

1. Hands on your knees, extend your spine and raise your shoulders up while inhaling deeply. Keeping your hands on your knees, round your back while exhaling. Repeat seven times.

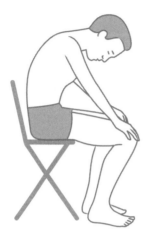

2. Hands on your knees, inhale while gently pushing your shoulders and head back, elongating your spine. Keeping your hands on your knees, round your back while exhaling. Repeat seven times.

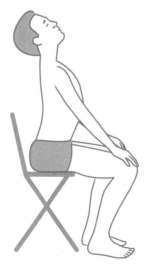

3. Regularly cross one leg on the other and hold your folded knee with one hand, the ankle of the bent leg with the other. Inhale while rounding your back and your spine. Relax while exhaling. Inhale while extending your back (imagine somebody is pulling you up by the hair!) then relax while exhaling. Repeat both exercises seven times each.

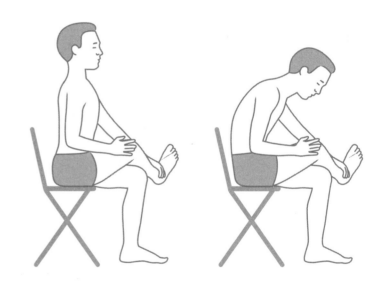

My cocooning space

 Sometimes, wisewoman recipes are surprising. For example, burdock can be used for an herbal tea or in an acne lotion! Below are a few go-to homemade remedies.

Acne

◎ Drop 1½ handful of burdock roots and leaves in 1 liter of boiling water. Steep for ten minutes. Apply on the face once a day for seven days.

Canker sores

◎ Three minutes a day, rinse your mouth with aloe vera juice. Also recommended for gingivitis and toothaches.

Bruises, burns, and sprains

◎ Sprinkle green clay on bruises and burns to speed up scarring. For sprains, use as a cataplasm kept in place by a bandage or a piece of cloth.

Cold sore

◎ Apply ice for forty-five minutes each day, two days in a row.

Dark circles

◎ Seep a tea bag. Let cool and apply on the eyes for twenty minutes.

Warts

◎ Gather fig tree leaves. Crush them to extrude their milky sap, which you will apply on the wart morning and evening for twenty-five days.

◎ Other recipe: hollow out an onion and place coarse salt in the cavity. Apply the liquid produced by the onion morning and evening for fifteen days.

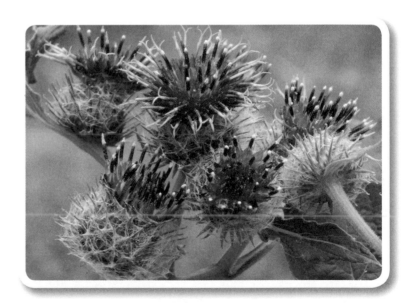

NATURE OFFERS RECIPES TO HEAL ALL COMMON ILLS.

My anti-stress moment

Once a week one needs to engage in sports to get rid of stress. It fosters toxin elimination and brings oxygen to your metabolism while regenerating and soothing your mind. This is not a marathon here, but rather a run or a brisk walk in true consciousness. Remember to wear clothes that let your body breathe and the right shoes.

1. Start by breathing to fire up your stomach-lungs engine and stretch. Legs apart, extend your left arm up and put your right hand on your right shin. Inhale/exhale several times. Switch sides.

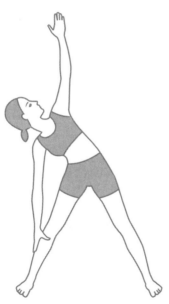

2. Lying on your back, grab your left knee with your right hand. Gently stretch your thigh while exhaling. Repeat seven times. Switch sides. If needed, use a cushion to prop up your buttocks.

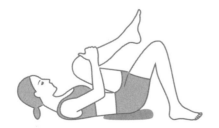

3. Sitting on the floor, back straight and legs bent, inhale. Exhale while bringing your head to your knee. Repeat seven times.

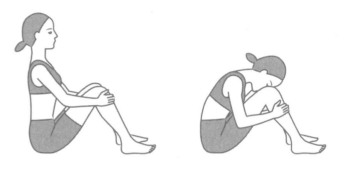

4. Always start by running slowly. Then accelerate and find your natural pace. Stay focused on your breath, which will regulate itself. If you don't call upon your mind and are simply experiencing your present physical state, you are showing respect to your body; you will experience harmony and your stress will diminish by itself.

5. Finally, bring your attention to painful or "no tension" zones: a kind look at your body fosters de-stress. Learn to talk to your body: consider its well-being and it will reciprocate.

My art therapy moment

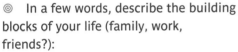 ## Develop your energies

◎ Staying in tune with your vital needs keeps you energized! Start by coloring the central star, symbol of your expanding energy. Continue towards the outside of the mandala using warm colors like red, orange, and yellow.

◎ In a few words, describe the building blocks of your life (family, work, friends?):

. . . .
. . . .
. . . .
. . . .
. . . .
. . . .
. . . .
. . . .
. . . .
. . . .
. . . .
. . . .
. . . .

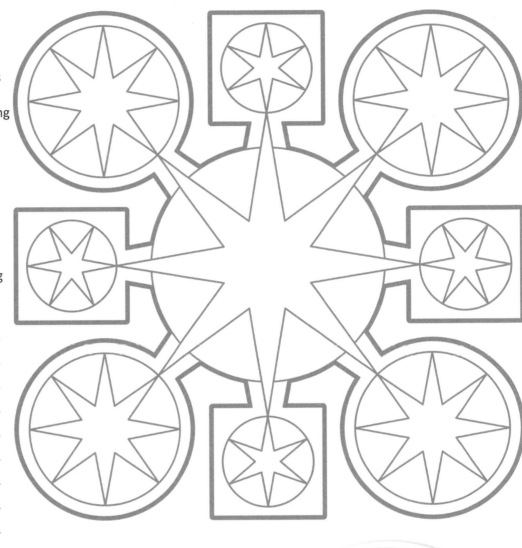

Meditate on this sentence:

Giving is a joy.
Giving of yourself
is the supreme joy.

Marie Valyère

Health Tip

Tap your forearms so as to stimulate and relax their muscles. These muscles are too often reduced to micro-movements (computer mouse, smartphone, etc.)

105

My path to well-being

Continue your joint training by gently working on your torso, knees, and ankles. Use a stable chair on which you can rest your foot without straining your leg.

1. Facing the chair, put your left foot flat on the seat. Left hand on your left hip, inhale while your torso pivots slowly to the right. Exhale, coming back to your original position. Repeat at least three times. Switch sides.

2. With your back to the chair, hands on your hips, put your left foot on the chair. Inhale while slightly bending your right knee. Come back to your original position while exhaling. Repeat at least three times. Switch sides.

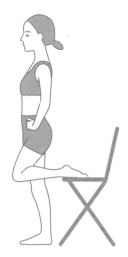

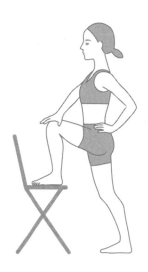

3. Sitting on the edge of the chair, extend your left arm back to reach the back of the chair. Bend your torso forward as you inhale. Exhale while coming back to your original position. Repeat at least three times. Switch sides.

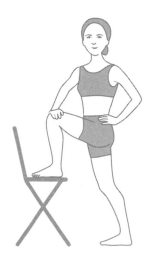

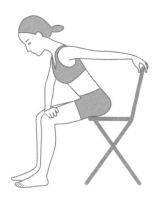

My cocooning space

Blenders are wonderful: they can purée everything from frozen fruits and ice cubes to fresh fruit and vegetables, with or without adding liquid. Enjoy energizing vitamin juices on demand all year round!

 Here are some ideas. Adapt to each season.

Cantaloupe-apricot

◎ ½ cubed cantaloupe, ½ cup of apricot nectar, 1 teaspoon of honey, and ½ cup of crushed ice.
◎ Mix until homogenous.

Orange-banana

◎ 1 cup of orange juice, ½ banana, ½ cup of vanilla yogurt, and ½ cup of crushed ice.
◎ Mix until homogenous.

Blueberries-grapes

◎ ½ cup of blueberries, 1 sliced banana, ½ cup of white grape juice, and ½ cup of crushed ice.
◎ Mix until homogenous.

Cranberry-lemon

◎ 1 liter of mineral water, 1 cup of cranberry juice, 1 sliced orange, 1 sliced lemon, and 1 cup of crushed ice.
◎ Mix until homogenous.

Kiwi-Honey

◎ 2 peeled kiwis, 1 tablespoon of honey.
◎ Mix until homogenous. Pour into a large glass and add mineral water and ice cubes.
◎ Drink immediately.

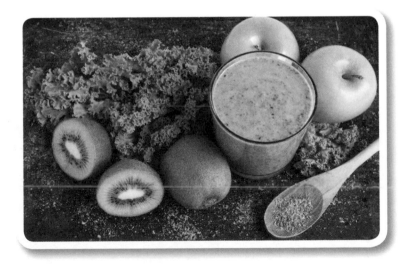

GET YOUR YEAR-ROUND VITAMINS IN ENERGIZING JUICES.

My anti-stress moment

Water is a very accessible vector of de-stress. It fosters quick relaxation and clears up dark moods or emotional states. Below are a few pointers for using water in all its forms.

Footbath

◎   Fill a dishpan with lukewarm water. Add a good handful of coarse salt.
◎   Let your feet soak for a few minutes: your kidneys will be revived and your mind soothed while you are getting rid of negative energies.

Shower

◎   Run lukewarm water. Place your showerhead above your head. Start with your nape. Then, alternate the distance of your showerhead to work on your scalp and feel the intensity of a direct natural massage.
◎   Aim directly above your kidneys. Change the distance of the showerhead to massage the suprarenal glands.
◎   Go down from your solar plexus to your lower stomach.
◎   Continue with your thighs, shins, and soles. Finish by going up each leg, which will stimulate your energy.

Drink

◎   First thing in the morning, drink a glass of bottled mineral or fresh water (it is better to alternate regularly), in order to cleanse your body from the work your cells have performed overnight.
◎   Avoid tap water, even filtered, which is magnetically dead!

Bath

◎   Baths are relaxing, but adding eleven ounces of coarse salt in your bathtub will alleviate stress, particularly if you feel "drained" after a long day's work with your team or with the public!
◎   Soak for at least twenty minutes. Immerse yourself several times.
◎   Finish with a shower and shampoo. De-stressed!

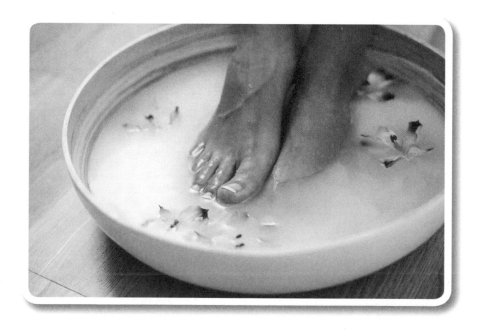

My art therapy moment

✏ Go from negative to positive!

◎ Art therapy is recommended when you feel caught in a whirlwind of negative thoughts, yours or those of people around you, carrying their gloominess and their pessimistic state of mind. In this case, think color and signs of joy: color the mandala, choosing soft or flashy colors. Make a point of avoiding black, brown, and dark purple.

◎ In a few words, describe the joys you like to experience:

. . . .

. . . .

. . . .

. . . .

. . . .

. . . .

. . . .

. . . .

. . . .

. . . .

. . . .

. . . .

. . . .

. . . .

. . . .

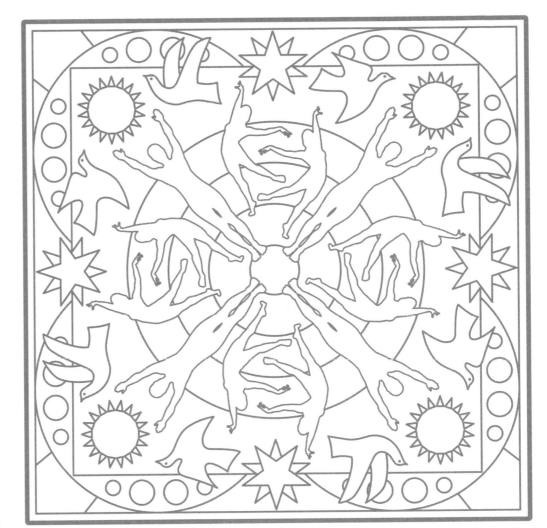

Meditate on this sentence:

The greatest pleasure in life is doing what people say you cannot do.

Walter Bagehot

Coaching Tip

Drink tea or herbal tea with happy red fruit notes. Also treat yourself to some chocolate. Bring sweetness to your life. . . .

My path to well-being

If you are sitting for most of the day, your lumbar muscles are probably strained. To relieve them, it is recommended to voluntarily work the muscles that stabilize your spine.

1. On all fours, look downward, your head aligned with your spine. Inhale while pushing your navel in and tightening perineum muscles (as if trying not to urinate), then exhale for about three seconds, keeping your perineum muscles tight. Repeat seven times.

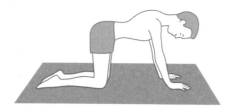 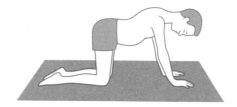

2. Sitting on your heels, place your palms on the floor behind you, fingers pointing away from you. Bring your right knee up, with your sole on the floor. Open the torso while inhaling and lifting your buttocks slightly. Feel the left thigh muscles stretching and the lower back working. Come back to your original position while exhaling. Repeat three times. Switch sides. Be gentle. This should not be painful.

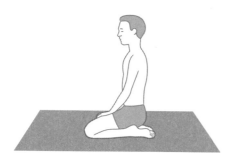 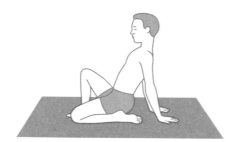 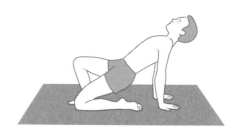

My cocooning space

Did you know that your intestines also encompass neurons, just like your heart and all your other organs? Unhealthy intestinal walls let toxins into your blood stream—therefore into your body—causing potentially grave problems.

Here is what you can do to maintain your intestines and your gut flora:

◎ Progressively give up refined grains, like white bread and white pasta. As a transition, favor semi-whole grains.

◎ Realize that improper cooking time destroys enzymes and vitamins.

◎ Do not consume too many uncooked fruits and vegetables. Their swift transit prevents the intestinal flora from restoring itself. Think about drinking a lot of water to keep your gut moist.

◎ Avoid stimulants like alcohol and coffee because they harden the intestinal mucus membrane.

◎ Too much animal protein produces putrefaction in your intestine.

◎ Leguminous plants like beans can cause fermentation when consumed too often.

◎ Spices can quickly irritate your colon.

◎ Clean all your fruit and vegetables before using them. Foods consumed raw have to be fresh (ground beef for steak tartar, fish for sushi, etc.)

Consult a dietician once or twice a year to get guidance on your food choices and information on their possible consequence on the organism.

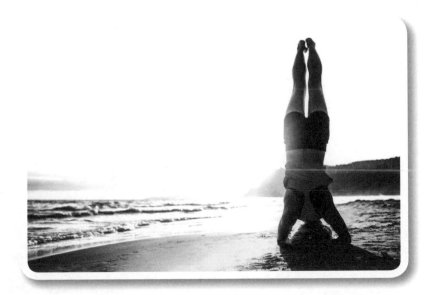

OUR IMMUNE SYSTEM IS THE BEST DEFENSE AGAINST STRESS.

My anti-stress moment

Being judgmental is a mental concept that generates lots of stress. This condition often becomes an obstacle to other views that go far beyond the simple duality of mental and emotional functioning. Hence frustrations, or worse, disregard!

Decide to meditate during your daily activities, while being a parent, a worker, a spouse. You will need to take a five-minute break each time:

1. While sitting down or walking, listen to your breath for a few moments. If your mind wanders, return to your breathing. If a thought comes to mind, refocus. Do this for five minutes.

2. Observe what is to your right and what is to your left without judging. Things happen, don't mind them! If someone brushes you, don't interpret. If somebody stares, let it go without thinking. Everything is acceptable, everything has a right to be, and, above all, to exist without you or beyond you.

3. Come back to your terrestrial responsibilities. By practicing this stepping back regularly, you will acquire a non-judgmental distance that will leave much more oxygen for you to fully live in your own present!

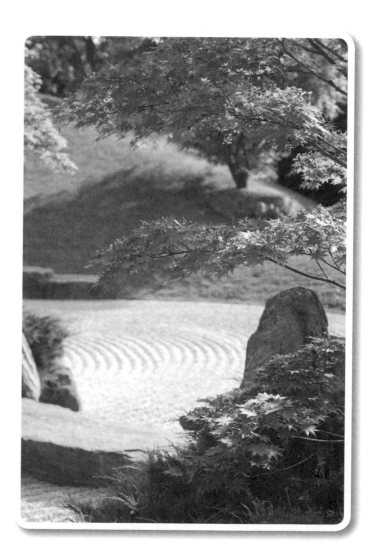

My art therapy moment

Letting go of your burdens

◎ In the lake, on top of the mountain, write words that evoke emotionally heavy "burdens." Below, in the ocean, note the ones that are synonymous with lightness.

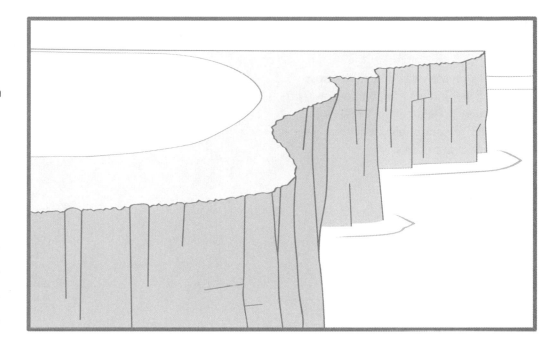

◎ Write joyous and positive sentences:

. . . .
. . . .
. . . .
. . . .
. . . .
. . . .
. . . .
. . . .
. . . .
. . . .
. . . .
. . . .
. . . .
. . . .
. . . .
. . . .
. . . .

Meditate on this sentence:

Average strength excites violence. Supreme strength elicits lightness.

Gilbert Keith Chesterton

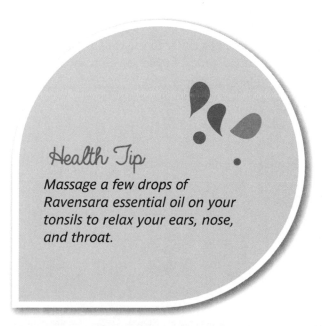

Health Tip

Massage a few drops of Ravensara essential oil on your tonsils to relax your ears, nose, and throat.

My path to well-being

If you are sitting down most of the day, make sure no part of your lower back is forgotten by practicing the following regularly.

1. Sitting on the edge of a chair, cross your hands behind your head and slowly lift your left knee while inhaling. Exhale while coming back to your original position. Repeat seven times. Switch sides.

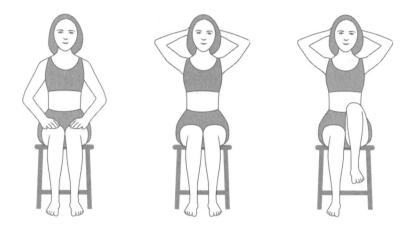

2. Facing a wall, feet parallel, palms on the wall, and arms extended, let your body lean forward. Feel how your body is aligned: your legs, then your spine, all the way to your head. Exhaling, get closer to the wall by flexing your arms a few times. Inhale as you come back to your original position.

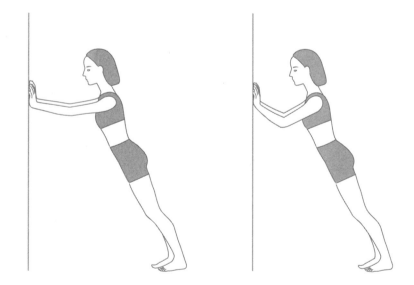

SPARE YOUR LOWER BACK, KEEP YOUR SPINE STRAIGHT.

My cocooning space

Bread is a cultural institution. Today, thanks to the fabulous bread machines available on the market, many families are making their own. Let us reiterate that—consumed on a regular basis—white flour irritates our bowels. Many of us even need to avoid gluten. Here are a few pointers on how to choose your flour and how to make great bread at home.

How to choose flour

◎   The French flour classification system is numeric. The smaller the number, the more refined the flour, i.e. the poorer in minerals: T65, T80, T110.

◎   In the United States, flour is divided into six categories: all-purpose flour, bread flour, cake flour, durum flour, high-gluten flour, pastry flour, and whole wheat flour.

Homemade whole wheat bread

◎   In a bowl, mix 16 ounces of organic, unbleached wheat flour (T110), 1 cup of bottled water, 0.7 ounces fresh yeast, and 2 teaspoons of salt.
◎   Knead about 10 minutes, until the dough is supple and not sticky. Make a ball, cover with a kitchen towel, and let rise for 30 minutes.
◎   Shape your bread. Let it rise for another 60 minutes. Place on a baking sheet. Bake for 45 minutes at 350 degrees F.

Gluten-free bread loaves

◎   Completely dissolve 1 teaspoon of salt in 12.5 cups of water. Add 1 tablespoon of butter to the salty water and warm up.
◎   In a bowl, mix 7 ounces of rice flour, 7 ounces of buckwheat flour, 2 tablespoons of almond powder, and 2 tablespoons of soy milk (or semi-skimmed cow milk).
◎   Add 2 tablespoons of leavening yeast to the warm, salty water. Mix with a wooden spoon and add 2 tablespoons of poppy seeds. Let rise 3 hours.
◎   Place in greased individual loaf baking dishes. Bake 20 minutes at 390 degrees F.

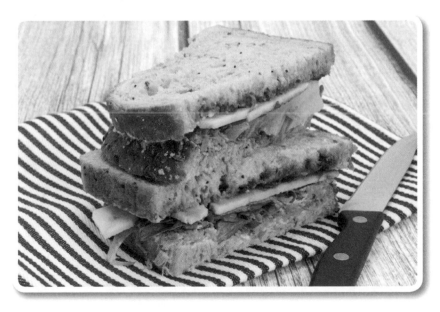

My anti-stress moment

Your brain emits thoughts constantly. An average of sixty thousand thoughts a day are generated by a natural and unconscious mechanism! The electric activity tires the brain and disturbs attention, particularly because 80 percent of these thoughts are recurring. This excess generates stress and its production wastes a lot of energy at the expense of vision, attention, and concentration.

Object focused meditation can teach us to focus on one object, one request at a time. It can be practiced anywhere, even at work. It slows down the electric rhythm of the brain and, consequently, stress. Here is how to structure a five-to-ten minute session. For best results, practice regularly (and twice a day!).

1. Simply concentrate on a common object, such as a notebook on your desk. Place it twenty-four inches away from you. Your hands are flat on your desk. Look at the bottom of the notebook. Concentrate on the notebook (thin or thick, square or rectangular, spiral or not, color, etc.). Do not analyze it, simply observe.

2. You will quickly note that your breath is already slower, more peaceful. During this short session, you should not think about anything else but what you see (the notebook). Every time a thought appears in your mind, refocus your attention on the notebook, its shape, its color, etc.

3. When you are totally focused on this notebook, totally invested in the present, your brain will be conscious of your surroundings and mentally available: you will be centered on the essential and not "lost" in your tiring thoughts!

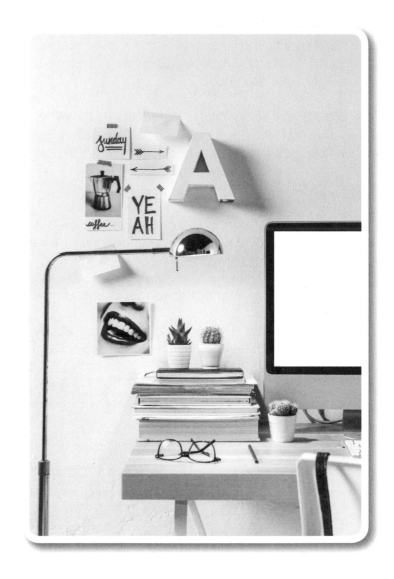

My art therapy moment

✏️ ## Expression mandala

◎ To solidify your meditation session, color this mandala as a focus object. The center is green, the rest evolves between yellow and orange, then light blue.

◎ Write a few soothing words that you could use during your meditation:

....
....
....
....
....
....
....
....
....
....
....
....
....
....
....
....
....
....
....

Meditate on this sentence:

Each one of us is responsible for expanding our inner peace so all of us can reach world peace.

Dalai Lama

Health Tip

To foster concentration, diffuse a few drops of Pettitgrain essential oil for a few minutes.

My path to well-being

Do you know the bear and the tree exercise? It's a simple and efficient way to relax the lower back while working the abdomen at the same time!

1. Your back against a wall, arms extended at a forty-five degree angle, bring your feet somewhat forward so as to let yourself slide down the wall. When you are low enough to sit in a chair, go back up again, your back always in contact with the wall. Use your abdominals, but also your hands and your arms. Repeat at least seven times. Take a few steps to restore full blood circulation.

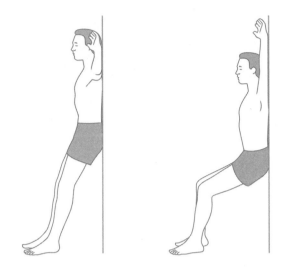

2. Lie on your back, soles touching the wall, arms away from the body, legs slightly apart and bent. Without moving your feet, simply bring your knees together and apart. Repeat two sequences of seven. Rest your feet on the floor and breathe calmly.

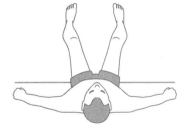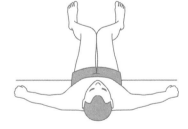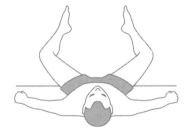

My cocooning space

 The whole family needs milk, so why not suggest a yogurt preparation and tasting session? Every one can participate and contribute to this simple and delicious recipe!!

You will need: 1 liter of whole milk (cow, sheep, or goat, the last two making more liquid yogurts), a yogurt maker or a pressure cooker (very easy to find second hand), 8 glass yogurt jars, a cooking thermometer, and 1 pack of yogurt starter culture for 8 yogurts (available in organic stores).

◎   Bring the milk to a boil. Let it cool down to 104 degrees F, checking with your thermometer.

◎   Flavor by adding 1 drop of lavender, lemon, mandarin, or grapefruit essential oil or 1 teaspoon of agar-agar to create a thicker yogurt.

◎   Add the yogurt starter packet and mix with a spatula. Pour in the glass yogurt jars.

◎   Bring ½ a liter of water to boil in your pressure cooker. Take it off the heat, place the yogurt in the hot water, and close hermetically. Let sit for 8 hours, then place in the refrigerator for 4 hours.

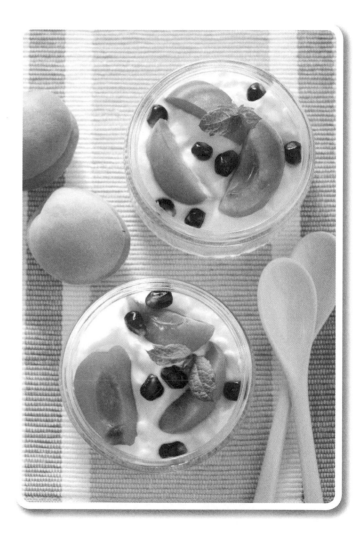

NATURALLY FLAVORED YOGURT ENERGIZES THE FAMILY!

My anti-stress moment

Writing workshop

Talking creates; it cures and allows us to express actions and events suffered passively. Stop for a moment to write a positive or even constructive sentence describing each of your life events, as far back as you can remember. It will be a way to keep you in a creative and dynamic thread that will erase the emotional or mental charge still tying you to the past. That charge often brings up baggage of deep sadness and explosive stress unrelated to the present. Repeat this exercise once a month for one year. Add a particularly positive event from each period of your life.

The chapters of my life

◎ 0 to 5 years old:

....

....

Positive event:

....

◎ 5 to 10 years old:

....

....

Positive event:

....

◎ 10 to 15 years old:

....

....

Positive event:

....

◎ 15 to 20 years old:

....

....

....

Positive event:

....

◎ 20 to 25 years old:

....

Positive event:

....

◎ 25 to 30 years old:

....

Positive event:

....

◎ 30 to 35 years old:

....

Positive event:

....

◎ 35 to 40 years old:

....

Positive event:

....

◎ 40 to 45 years old:

....

Positive event:

....

My art therapy moment

✎ Becoming aware of what you already have

◎ Use this Mind Map to discover the positives life has already dealt you. Write the name of a person close to you (or glue in his or her picture) in each cloud surrounding the central bubble. Choose people who seem to have accompanied you during difficult times. Use an arrow to link each event to one or several people. You can actually see and become aware of the help you have already received.

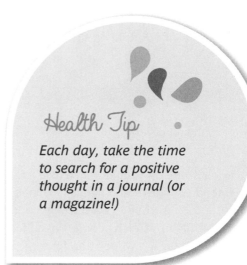

Health Tip

Each day, take the time to search for a positive thought in a journal (or a magazine!)

◎ In a few words, unpack the word "positive":

. . . .

. . . .

. . . .

. . . .

. . . .

. . . .

. . . .

. . . .

. . . .

. . . .

. . . .

. . . .

. . . .

. . . .

. . . .

Positive

Meditate on this sentence:

He who knows others is wise. He who knows himself is enlightened

Lao-Tseu

My path to well-being

We now introduce you to a series of simple and ancient poses, useful to align every tiny muscle that stabilizes every single vertebrae of your spine.

1. Lying prone on your stomach (use a towel if needed), extend your arms and hands in front of you, thumbs toward the ceiling. Your legs are straight and slightly apart. While breathing in, stretch your left hand forward and your right leg backward. Stay in this position for three seconds. Slowly release the stretch while exhaling. Do the same with your left leg and right arm. Repeat seven times, alternating sides.

2. Roll on your back and repeat the previous stretch, seven times on each side. Use a towel under your head if need be. Finish by taking a rest, arms along your body and eyes shut.

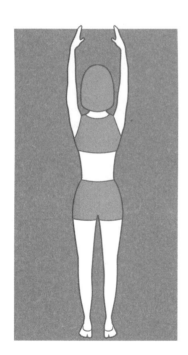 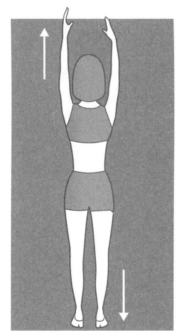 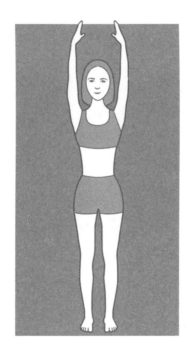 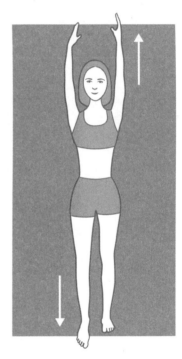

WORKING YOUR SPINE RESTORES YOUR ENERGY.

My cocooning space

 Homemade jams are a good source of fruit for every one to enjoy during winter, and they are great to share!

You will need: between 1 and 2 pounds of brown sugar for 2 pounds of fruit, agar-agar (a natural thickening agent), and lemon juice for stabilizing fruit color, preventing sugar crystallization, and improving jellification.

Strawberry jam

◎ Mix 2 pounds of cleaned strawberries with 1.8 pounds of sugar and the juice of 1 lemon. Let sit overnight.
◎ The next day, strain the strawberries and reserve them. Bring the juice to a boil for 10 minutes, stirring occasionally. Add the strawberries and cook under low heat for 10 more minutes. Add 2 teaspoons of agar-agar and continue cooking for 3 minutes.
◎ Pour the jam into glass jars, close, and sterilize for 2 hours.

Rhubarb jam

◎ Chop 2.8 pounds of clean rhubarb. Add 2 pounds of sugar and the juice of 1 lemon. Let sit overnight in a cool place.

◎ In the morning, strain the rhubarb and reserve it. Heat the juice, add the rhubarb, and allow to simmer for about 10 minutes, skimming away the foam as needed. Add 2 teaspoons of agar-agar and cook 5 more minutes.

◎ Pour the jam into glass jars, close, and sterilize for 2 hours.

◎ Take the time to let the fruit soak overnight. You will taste the difference!

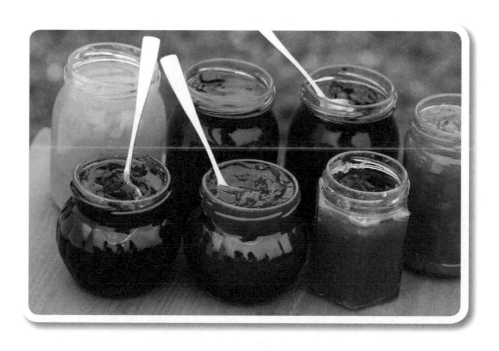

Group exchange

Organizing a well-being workshop is a simple and pleasant way to bring a group of people together. Breathing is the most commonly appreciated topic. Give a free course of de-stressing through breathing and you will have facilitated a useful meeting of the minds around a topic of interest! Here is a basic program. Each participant is encouraged to do what is available to him or her at the moment.

Feel your whole body breathing

1. Exhale fully. Inhale through the nose and inflate your stomach as much as possible. The diaphragm is lowered and compresses the abdominal organs. Without letting air out of your stomach, open your thorax so air fills the medium level of the lungs. Then, lift up your shoulders to let the air in the upper level of your lungs. Keep the air in (or not) while moving your head from side to side as if saying no. This opens the carotid artery that irrigates the brain. Slowly exhale through the nose: first the shoulders, then the thorax, and finally the stomach. Repeat twice.

2. Arms extended in front of you, bring them up as you inhale (no arms above the head before full inhalation). Bring the arms down as you exhale. Repeat three times.

3. Fists against your torso, inhale while pushing on the middle of your chest. Let the air explode out as your two fists open in front of you. Repeat three times.

4. For a collective meditation see weeks two or four of this book. Finish the session with silent relaxation on the floor.

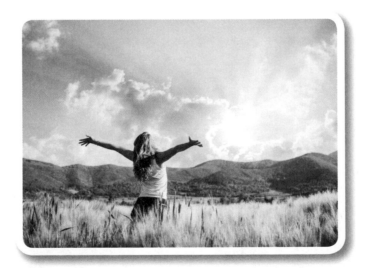

MEET BEYOND THE VERBAL WHILE BREATHING TOGETHER.

Group creativity

In a clearly defined framework, a mandala stimulates the expression of an original form of creativity channeled through coloring, photographs, or colored sand (ground mandalas, for example). Leading a group creativity session means that, to publicize a cause, support a project, or introduce an idea, you organize an afternoon meeting at your home or a community event during which you provide the necessary materials: paper, felt-tip color markers, and one mandala per participant.

◎ Example: Your group wishes to publicize the restoration of an old water well. At the center of the mandala would be a photograph of the well. On the rest of the page, concentric circles in which each participant inputs objects and colors.

◎ Give two clear instructions. To experience how a mandala facilitates concentration, the participant starts from the center and evolves towards the edges of the page. To experience how a mandala brings relaxation, the participant starts from the outside circle and progresses towards the center.

◎ It behooves the leader to establish a matrix that can be reproduced and modified, if need be.

◎ Each mandala can be posted, entered in a contest, or published in a local newsletter. It is important to offer this type of activity each year. Local communities appreciate peaceful and creative group activities during which neighbors can meet.

◎ Various local groups organize "mandala of the year" events.

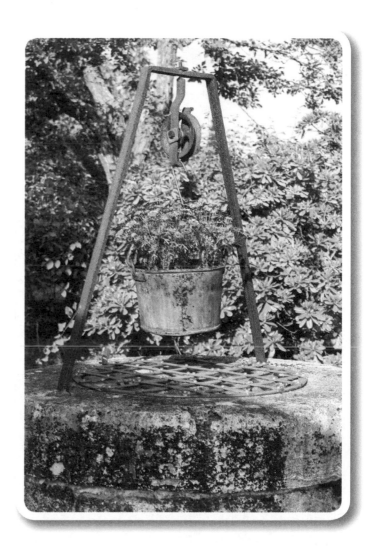

Art therapy collective

Talking groups organically combine de-stressing and art, a very natural duo. You will need an expression room, bars of clay, and a symbolic staff called a "talking stick" or "speaker's staff" to keep with the indigenous tradition of the Northwestern American coast peoples.

All the participants sit in a circle, if possible on a cushion. On the floor, in front of each one, is a piece of material with some clay and some newspapers for the participants to wipe their hands with or crumple instead of clay.

◎ A large garbage can is placed in the center of the circle.

◎ Sitting in the center, holding the talking stick, the organizer of the activity announces the topic (either chosen ahead of time or drawn out of a hat). Examples: nervousness, resentment, anger, melancholy, etc.

◎ First, everyone thinks about the topic and works the clay silently during three minutes.

◎ The organizer asks for comments on the topic and gives the first person the talking stick. As long as the person is holding the talking stick, everybody listens! The stick is passed back to the organizer and on to the next person, etc.

◎ When everyone has spoken, the organizer asks the group to resume kneading their clay, then to put it in the central garbage can with the determination to close the case and move on.

◎ Another topic might be tackled next. At the end of every session the organizer asks participants to exchange friendly greetings, then cordially thanks all the participants!

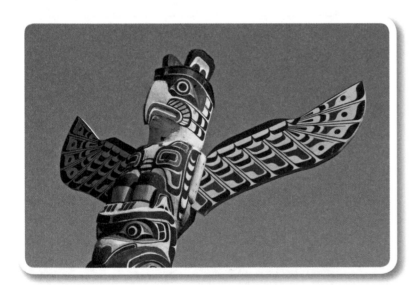

LISTENING TO ONE OF US BRINGS RESPECT TO ALL OF US.

My anti-stress moment

Compassion is an extremely powerful feeling. It is because you listen to others and understand their problems that you progressively become mindful of what irks you in this world because you don't have a solution. Compassion generates self-valorization and self-respect. Here is how to develop compassion through meditation.

1. Sit with your back straight. For a few moments, breathe calmly as you look in front of you. Think about an event or a person who is going through a rough patch.

2. Close your eyes and imagine you are with that person, smiling or, at least, experiencing positive feelings, kind thoughts.

3. Imagine the person telling you the reasons for his or her current difficulties. Imagine that you are responding with words of peace and fraternal love, providing comfort. After you experience all these feelings, let the person go, totally changed, peaceful, smiling, and relieved. Wave and peacefully get back to your business.

Try to adopt this mindset that, as you will soon realize, also opens your heart.

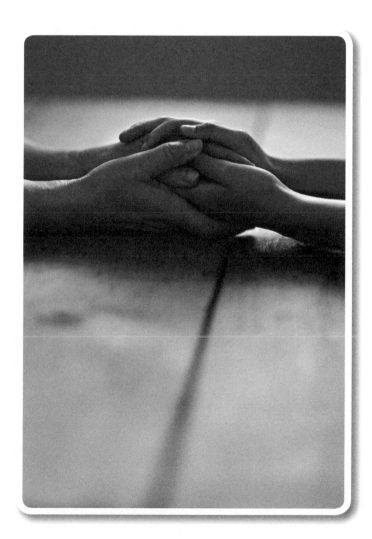

My art therapy moment

Selfless presents

◎ Use a different color for each leaf and imagine that you are giving the leaves to specific people who need the attention.

◎ Write a few comforting words that you would like to tell somebody you know:

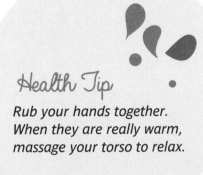

Meditate on this sentence:

Everything you want is waiting for you. Everything you want wants you back. But you have to get up and get it.

Jack Canfield

Health Tip

Rub your hands together. When they are really warm, massage your torso to relax.

My path to well-being

Still on our path to well-being, strengthening your back requires you to focus on all your vertebrae-supporting muscles, which are weakened by sitting down most of the day.

1. Sitting on the edge of your chair, place a thick towel between your knees. Extend your arms out shoulder-height while slowly breathing in. Turn your palms towards the sky, thumbs pushed in, abs engaged. Keep the position while slowly breathing out, still holding the towel between your knees. Feel your shoulder blades and the muscles along your spine work! Be gentle. Repeat seven times, progressively holding the position longer before coming back to your original position.

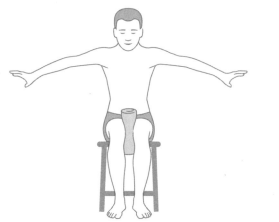
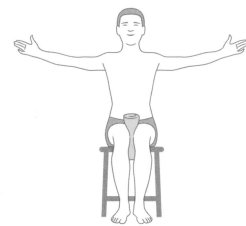

2. Still sitting on the edge of your chair, clasp your hands together and interlock your fingers; inhale while bringing your hands above your head; gently stretch your hands towards the ceiling, keeping your back straight. Exhale while bringing your arms down. Repeat seven times.

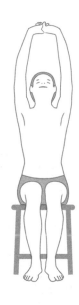

My cocooning space

Over the last couple of years many people have switched from coffee to tea, even though the boost is quite different. Tea has virtues for the body and mind, but because theanine is a stimulant, it might affect your stomach or even your digestion. Because it diminishes iron absorption, it is not advisable to drink tea with a meal. Here are a few tips on how to choose and prepare tea.

Steeping times

During brewing, theanine diffuses in the cup, followed by the tannins, which neutralize the effect of theanine on the body.
◎ For a mildly stimulating tea, steep 1 to 2 minutes.
◎ For a mildly stimulating tea with a strong taste, steep 3 to 5 minutes.
◎ For a light theanine-free tea, pour water in a teapot and discard. Pour water anew and steep 2 minutes.

Choice of teas

◎ Black tea (India, China): tannic, rich flavor, high theanine content. Steep 3 to 4 minutes.
◎ Dark black Pu'ehr tea (China): slightly sweet, medium theanine content. Steep 3 to 4 minutes.
◎ Dark smoked black tea (China): smoked wood flavor, medium theanine content. Steep 4 to 5 minutes.
◎ Green tea (China, Japan, India): fresh or fruity flavor, mild theanine content. Steep 3 to 5 minutes.
◎ White tea (China): subtle aromas, not tannic, low theanine content. Steep 10 to 12 minutes.
◎ Rooibos, or "red tea" (South Africa): mild, not tannic, theanine free. Steep 5 to 10 minutes.

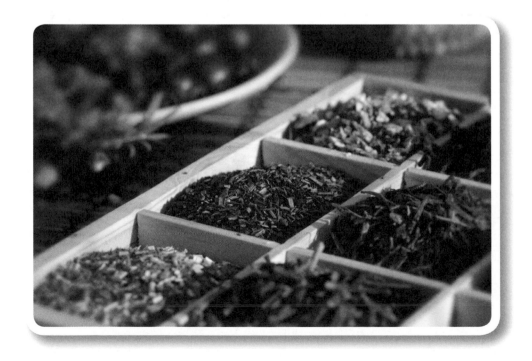

My anti-stress moment

Stress interferes with our attention and compassion in such a way that all of us tend to forget the positive moments we live every day. It is essential to train our mind to note the constructive. You only need a few minutes, once in the morning and once in the afternoon.

◎   You can train on your way to work or to your first appointment. For example, quietly focus your attention on croissants in the pastry shop window. Smile. Mental note to self: "croissants and smile." Then you walk past an adorable child. Mental note: "adorable child." If the weather is nice, look up and note: "blue sky, mild, and pleasant," etc.

This simple exercise calms your mind, opening a pleasant window to the people and world around you.

◎   Apply this method to your work environment or during meetings. For example, compassionately look at your colleague, use little details to feel peaceful while the rest of the group is tense. It could be a poorly knotted tie, a bored face . . . Learn to use the moment to create space and oxygen in your brain.

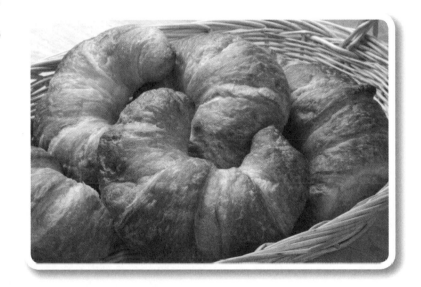

With time, you will realize that when you step back, stress goes away. You can find positive and pleasant moments in every day situations if you are attentive to the numerous little details of each moment of your day.

BEING POSITIVE ALSO MEANS STAYING CONSTRUCTIVE!

My art therapy moment

✏️ Very simple pleasures

◎ Relax while coloring each little detail with a different color (if possible) so as to create a multicolor owl, a carnival owl!

◎ Write a few words related to sharing and celebration:

....
....
....
....
....
....
....
....
....
....
....
....
....
....
....
....
....
....
....
....

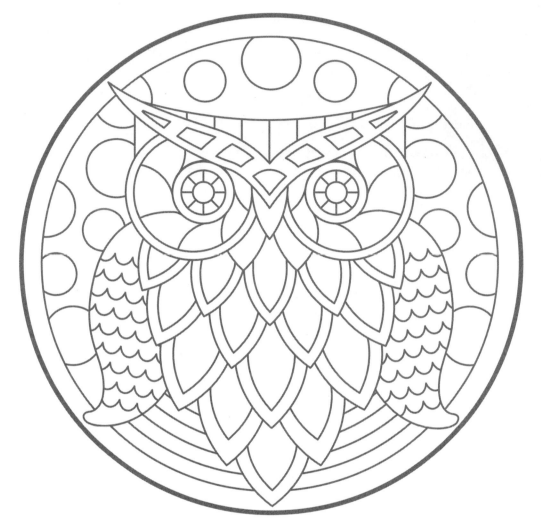

Meditate on this sentence:

Happiness is a secret joy that is lived in a dream.

Robert Lalonde

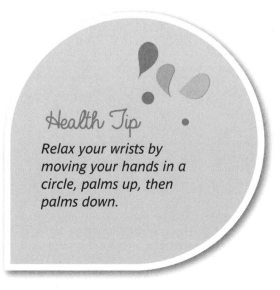

Health Tip

Relax your wrists by moving your hands in a circle, palms up, then palms down.

132

My path to well-being

To work the arch of your foot and make sure it stabilizes your body as much as it should, repeat the following simple exercise three times.

1. Bring your right arm up and your left foot up. Readjust your balance by slightly shifting your body. Let your right arch "work" and stabilize your body. It also forces your spine to stretch and your hips to gently engage.

2. Bring your foot to the floor, your arm along your body. Switch sides.

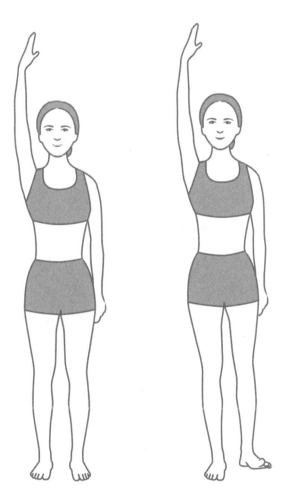

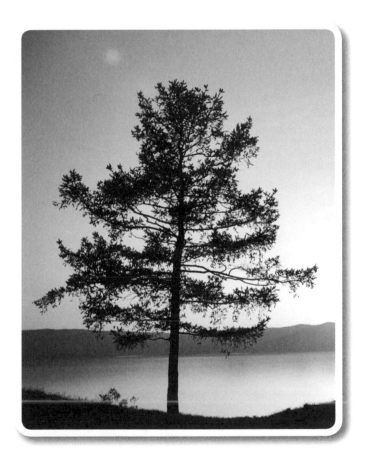

POSTURAL BALANCE RELIEVES YOUR STRESS.

My cocooning space

Being attentive to your well-being is but one stage on the path to happiness. We all need to learn to take care of ourselves. Nobody else can do it for you. Here are a few essential oils. They can be used alone or together to combine their action.

◎ Against deep sadness, diffuse a few drops of bergamot: this revitalizing essential oil is fresh and strengthens your desire to change your mood.

◎ If you are really unhappy or have just heard bad news, think about diffusing Neroli for a few minutes. Particularly efficient to calm anger.

◎ Bergamot and Neroli can be mixed, especially in the case of a panic attack.

◎ Add ylang-ylang to the previous two oils: its fruity hints efficiently relax the brain by dissipating negative thoughts.

◎ Lavender oil is antiseptic. Used alone, it purifies people's negativity and irritating smoke, or accompanies transitions in the course of the day.

◎ Lavender reinforces the effect of the three previous essential oils.

◎ Mandarin is used for its calming quality. Its sweet smell immediately brings joyous memories of fruit, cuddles, and childhood. It also induces sleep.

◎ Lemon reinforces your brain and your concentration.

◎ Lemon and mandarin create a delicious citric aroma, useful against mild anxiety.

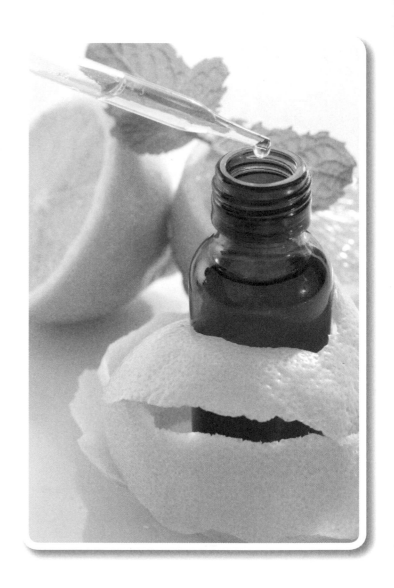

My anti-stress moment

When you know you are going to have a long day, do a "run through" the day beforehand. Then, apply these very simple anti-stress steps. Preventively defusing the charge of the upcoming situation frees some energy to better manage the day's tension.

The day before

◎ Plan a dinner that will be pleasant but low in protein and dairy products, avoiding the possible extra psychological burden of a difficult digestion.

◎ Spend the evening watching TV. Stay away from violent movies or stimulating shows!

On the morning

◎ If you don't have enough time for a relaxing shower, use the hand shower to massage your whole body in circular movements and harmonize your energy.

◎ Have a whole-grain breakfast: the slow sugar will hold you until lunch. Take some hazelnuts or almonds along as a pick me up!

◎ If using public transportation, breathe calmly, making sure your arches are firmly planted on the floor. If you can look down, visualize yourself in total control at work, energetic and efficient!

During the day

◎ As soon as you can, take one or two minutes to meditate, only observing what is around you, without specific thoughts. Take a mini-break to isolate yourself from the general turmoil and disengage from your direct environment. Listen to your needs. Need something to drink? Sit up to be more comfortable?

◎ Save some time to recharge, even if it means having lunch alone to avoid sad or over-excited discussions. If at all possible, escape five minutes out of every hour to reconnect with yourself.

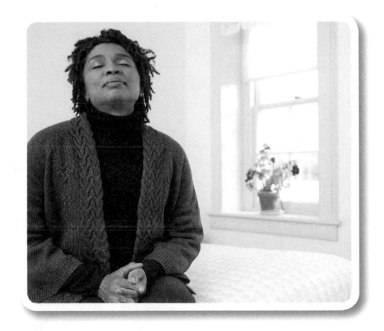

TO AVOID POSSIBLE TENSIONS, SET SIMPLE PREVENTIVE MARKERS.

My art therapy moment

✏️ Retreat in your own bubble

◎ Before important meetings or before making an important decision, it is useful and pleasant to take time to re-energize. Here is a mandala comprised of five possible universes; try to choose a specific dominant color for each one.

Health Tip

As you color, take short breaks. On the edge of your chair, stretch your back, arms up, nape slightly back.

◎ In a few words, list what evokes relaxation and escape:

. . . .

. . . .

. . . .

. . . .

. . . .

. . . .

. . . .

. . . .

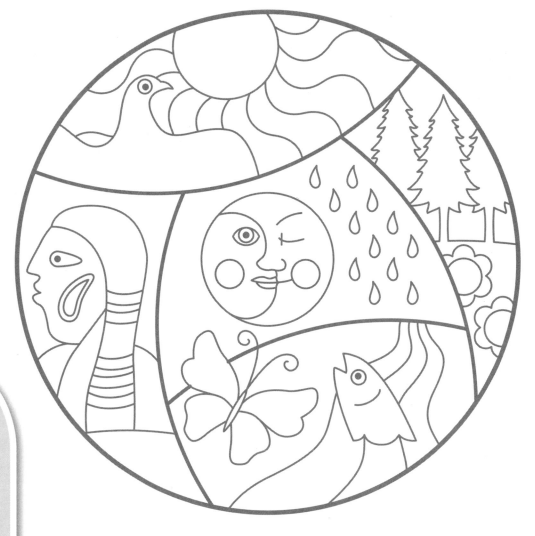

Meditate on this sentence:

Each step must be an objective.

Jacques Chirac

136

My path to well-being

Aligning your hips/spine/nape can be done on the floor. As an added bonus, you will work your pectorals and abs. Be gentle and progressive. This new approach to the infamous push-up still works the whole muscular mass! Progress at your own rhythm: start with three repetitions, then four, and so on.

1. Lie prone on your stomach, hands flat on each side of your face, elbows bent, knees and toes on the floor.

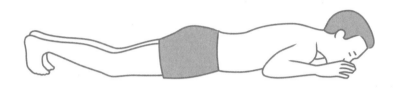

2. Supporting yourself on your forearms and fists, lift your torso up.

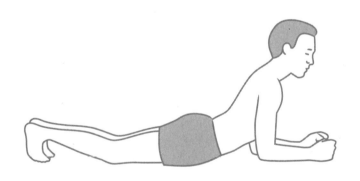

3. Slowly lift your hips up, without bending your back, knees still on the floor.

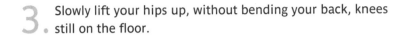
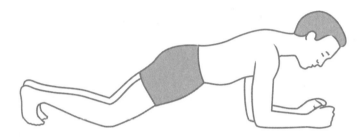

4. Lift your knees so your back is aligned with your extended legs. Hold the position a few seconds, your abs engaged.

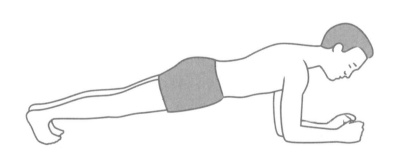

5. Reverse the movement to come back to the initial position.

My cocooning space

 Feuilles de brick (available at your supermarket or on line) or Phyllo dough are the basis of quick and delicious meals. Here are some ideas you can adapt to taste.

Egg Bricks

You will need: 8 *feuilles de brick,* 4 eggs, 2 zucchinis, 3.5 ounces of garlic cream cheese, 2 tablespoons of vegetable oil, some parsley, salt, and pepper.

1. Unroll 1 *feuille de brick.* Slather it with oil. Repeat for the other seven.

2. Rinse the zucchinis but do not peel them. Grate them or use your vegetable peeler to cut ribbons. Make a zucchini bed with a nest in the middle. Add salt and pepper to taste. Add pieces of cheese. Break one egg in the nest.

3. Bring the corners of the *feuilles de brick* in to create a pocket and place on an oiled baking sheet. Bake at 360 degrees F for 8 minutes or until the *feuilles de brick* start to get brown. Serve with fresh bread to dip in the yoke.

Spinach Bricks

You will need: 4 large *feuilles de brick,* ½ pound of young spinach leaves, ½ pound of raw and peeled shrimp, 1 avocado, 1 orange, 1 lemon, 1 red onion, 1 cucumber, 1 clove of garlic, 2 tablespoons of finely chopped Italian parsley, 4 tablespoons of olive oil, salt, and pepper.

1. Wash and drain the spinach. Peel and slice the avocado.

2. Press the juice of ½ orange and ½ lemon. Peel the other halves and cut them into thin slices.

3. Peel the cucumber and make ribbons with your vegetable peeler, avoiding the seeds in the center.

4. Peel and thinly cut the onion.

5. Place some spinach, cucumber, lemon, orange, avocado, and shrimp on the *feuilles de brick.* Fold to make pockets. Bake at 360 degrees F for 10 minutes.

6. In a bowl, mix the orange and lemon juices, salt, pepper, garlic, and parsley. Emulsify with the olive oil.

7. When they are ready, partially open the pockets, season them with the emulsified sauce and a sprinkle of chopped onion.

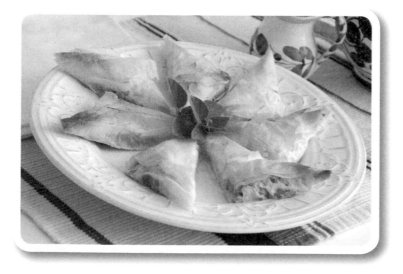

My anti-stress moment

Below are a few tips on how to use art to de-stress when you need to. Use this page now; you can use any sheet of paper when you want to repeat the exercise.

◎   De-stressing immediately: draw small balloons and fill them with dots, using the tip of a pen.

◎   Dissipating tension: draw spirals, narrow at the bottom, wide at the top.

◎   Breathing better: thin strokes at the bottom of the page, wide going up.

◎   Suffocating: draw two side-by-side vertical lines. Connect the two lines back and forth, going towards the top and the bottom of the page.

◎   Lacking energy to make yourself heard: draw ten exclamation points or ten small crosses with a point at the center.

◎   Relaxing and escaping: draw half curves open towards the top of the page. Add small shapes inside the curves, or simply scribble.

◎   Restoring energy: draw vertical lines starting from the same central point.

◎   Bringing joy: draw fireworks, like blooming flowers.

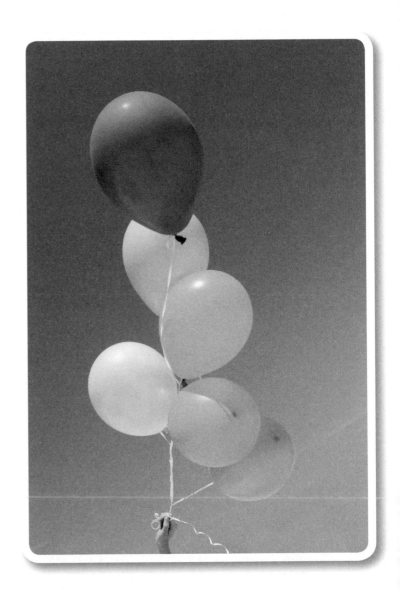

CONSCIOUS DRAWING RELEASES INTERNAL TENSIONS.

My art therapy moment

✏️ Escape in a fairy tale

◎ Supernatural worlds offer an escape from your day-to-day life. Color this fairy tale image with soft and peaceful colors.

◎ Write a few words that conjure up the peacefulness of children's tales:

. . . .

. . . .

. . . .

. . . .

. . . .

. . . .

. . . .

. . . .

. . . .

. . . .

. . . .

. . . .

. . . .

. . . .

. . . .

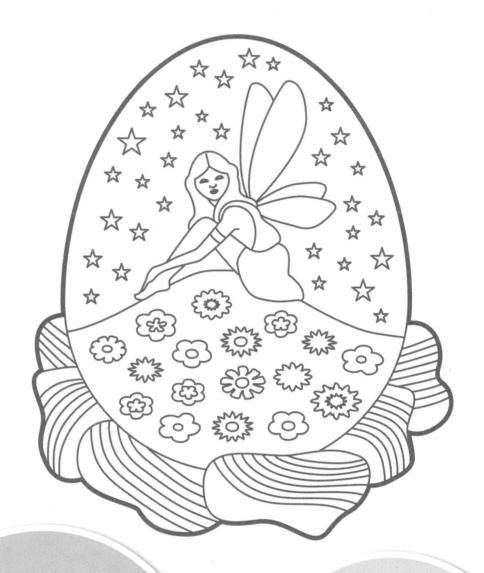

Meditate on this sentence:

When the first baby laughed for the first time, the laughter shattered into a million pieces that scattered everywhere. This is how the fairies were born.

James Barrie

Health Tip

In the evening, welcome sleep by diffusing a few drops of orange or grapefruit essential oils in your bedroom.

My path to well-being

Working on one's balance complements motor skills and body spatiality. The exercises below force your brain to use all your senses to find the right movement; they are a way to remain in the moment, feel your body, and find relaxation! Start with only one side of your body, then the other. Repeat three times.

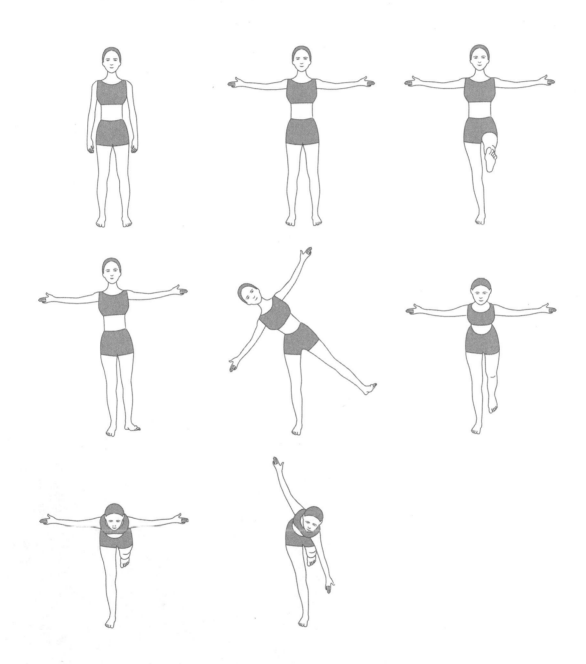

SPATIAL MOTOR SKILLS BRING YOU BACK INTO THE NOW.

My cocooning space

 Nothing is simpler than making pleasant and natural hair products for the whole family!

Marseille soap shampoo

1. Place ½ cup of dry or fresh rosemary in an airproof container. Pour 12.7 ounces of hot water, cover, and steep for 20 minutes.

2. Filter and add 3 tablespoons of Marseille soap shavings and 2 teaspoons of sesame oil. Stir and keep in a plastic bottle.

Nourishing algae conditioner

1. In a small dish, mix 1 teaspoon of powdered Iziki algae with 4.5 ounces of distilled water.

2. Massage on towel-dried hair. Protect your hair with a towel and keep for 10 minutes. Rinse with cold water.

Hair revitalizer

1. In a small container, mix ¼ cup of neutral powdered henna with ½ cup of plain yogurt until homogenous.

2. Apply on towel-dried hair. Protect your hair with a towel and keep for 20 minutes. Rinse with cold water.

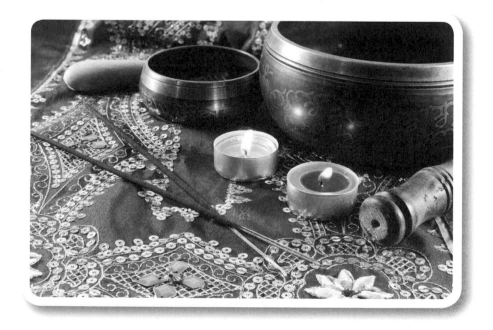

My anti-stress moment

De-stressing is also feeling free to say what we think and to write what we would like to do in our wildest dreams! Below is an expression forum: you can say everything, the worst and the best, the shameful and the strange, what you wouldn't dare tell anybody! We suggest a few themes, but feel free to add more.

Things I want to say

....
....
....
....
....
....
....

Things I can't disclose

....
....
....
....
....
....
....

Silliest things I want to do

....
....
....
....
....
....
....

Other

....
....
....
....
....
....

FREE SOME MENTAL SPACE: SAY WHAT IS ON YOUR MIND.

My art therapy moment

✏️ Relaxation and de-stressing

◎ While coloring, the mind transcends mental structures of representation, demonstration, and cohesion. Art therapy enables the subject to override all frameworks, so let your hair down and express anything with enchanting colors! Then, with the tip of a pen, prick the balloons to make them explode!

◎ Write a few "out-there" words that you find particularly amusing:

. . . .

. . . .

. . . .

. . . .

. . . .

. . . .

. . . .

. . . .

. . . .

. . . .

. . . .

. . . .

. . . .

. . . .

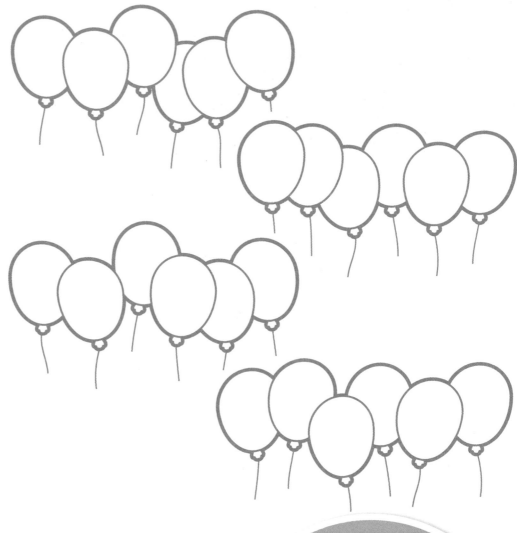

Meditate on this sentence:

Answers rarely establish the truth. A series of questions do.
Daniel Pennac

Health Tip

Standing or sitting, give slow-motion air punches, breathing slowly to de-stress.

My path to well-being

Conscious breathing and moving stimulates the flow of energy in the body. Here is a first path you should practice, gently, at least three times a week, repeating each exercise three times.

Lungs

Hands behind your back, thumbs locked, breathe in while extending your arms and lowering your upper body parallel to the floor.

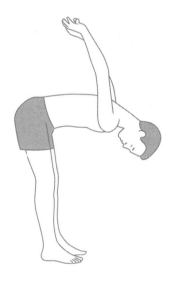

Spleen and stomach

Sitting on your soles, place your hands behind you, fingers pointing away from you. Breathe in while lifting your hips; breathe out coming back down.

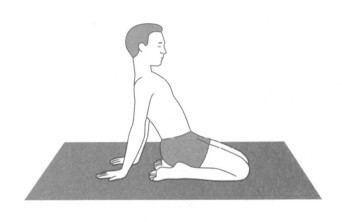

Solar Plexus (or Celiac plexus)

Place the index and the middle finger of both hands on your torso, where your ribs start (solar plexus). Breathe in and out slowly while gently pushing your fingers into your abdomen.

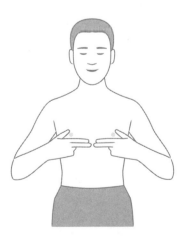

Bladder and kidneys

Sitting, legs and arms extended, palms facing out, bend forward pushing your shoulders forward and your head down. Breathe calmly a few times and feel the stretch of the lower back and kidneys. Come back to your original position.

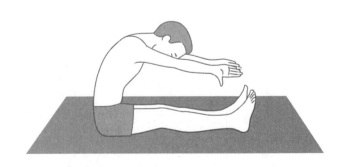

My cocooning space

 We all have experienced intellectual fatigue. Below we suggest a few simple remedies. Repeat them regularly so you are never without them! Treatments usually run three weeks.

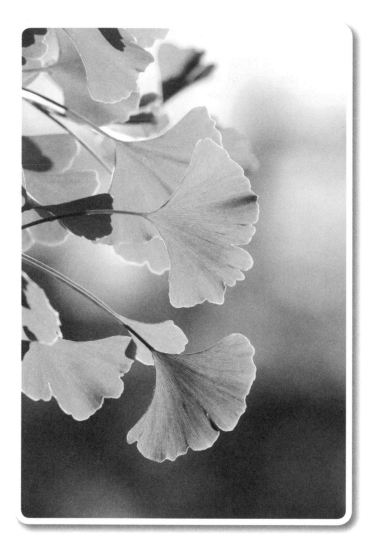

Ginkgo biloba

◎ Very efficient against fear of the blank page! Pleasant to drink as an infusion. Steep 0.3 ounces in 1 liter of boiling water for 10 minutes. Drink three cups a day.

Fatty fish

◎ If you need to enhance your intellectual performance, eat fatty fish (salmon, mackerel, and sardines) up to three times a week. Omega-3 rich krill oil is also available as a food complement.

Asparagus, wheat germ, lentils, watercress, and chervil

◎ Rich in folic acid, known to improve memory!

Nettles

◎ Whether in a capsule or as vegetable sap diluted in water, they provide iron and minerals and regenerate the mind.

YOUR FOOD INTAKE AFFECTS YOUR BRAIN TOO.

My anti-stress moment

De-stressing can also be done in emergency mode. Some immediate maneuvers exist, designed to avoid panic and incoherent reactions. They might not always be inconspicuous, but sometimes there is no other solution.

1. Make fists with both hands and place them on your chest. Inhale, while progressively increasing the pressure. Count to three and project your fists forward, arms extended, exhaling violently like a cork popping. Empty your lungs. Repeat three times.

2. Elbows at your side and fingers interlocked, swiftly rub your palms one against the other, particularly the pads at the bottom of your thumbs, until they become very hot. At the same time, inhale and exhale slowly. Your mind will calm down and your stress recede.

3. Stomach self-massage: move both your palms in clockwise circles while inhaling and exhaling normally.

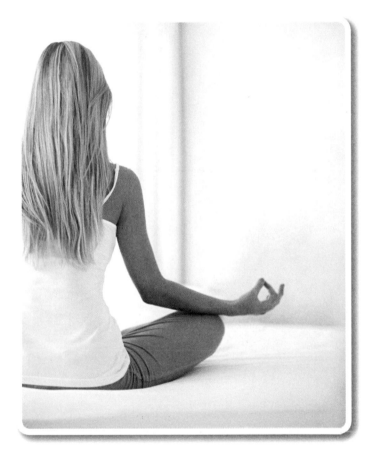

HEART RATE INCREASE? USE DE-STRESS MANEUVERS.

My art therapy moment

✏️ **Defining your future**

◎ Color this tree and the path to its right: what can you add that would symbolize a shining future? You can choose to draw or glue in meaningful images.

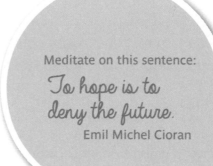

◎ In a few words, explain the above choices:

. . . .
. . . .
. . . .
. . . .
. . . .
. . . .
. . . .
. . . .
. . . .
. . . .
. . . .
. . . .
. . . .
. . . .
. . . .
. . . .
. . . .
. . . .
. . . .
. . . .
. . . .
. . . .

Health Tip

Bring together the thumb and the index finger of both your hands, close your eyes, and breathe a few moments in order to remain focused and relaxed.

148

My path to well-being

To continue maintaining our meridians, here is an easy path that you can practice at home between two activities. Logical after week thirty-six!

Liver and gallbladder

Sitting on the floor, cross your arms and bring your hands on your knees, pushing them down without forcing too much. Inhale and exhale while gently lowering your torso, emptying your lungs.

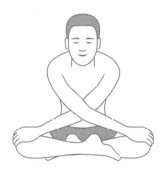 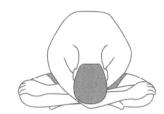

Heart

Sitting on the floor, join your soles together and hold them with your hands; lower your torso as much as available to you while breathing calmly. Feel your heart rate slow down.

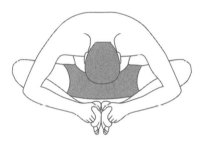

Intestines

Standing up, palms on your kidneys, bring your back to a 45 degree angle while exhaling. Hold the position and breathe in and out at your own rhythm.

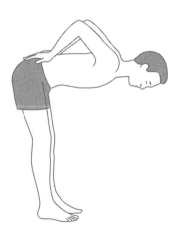

COORDINATED MOVEMENTS MAINTAIN YOUR ORGANS.

My cocooning space

In the city, not only are we exposed to traffic pollution outdoors, but we are also susceptible to the indoor pollution caused by materials and cleaning products. Take remedial measures by making your own people and environment-friendly cleaning products.

All-purpose cleaner

◎ For 1 liter of cleaner: 1 liter of hot water, 1 tablespoon of baking soda, 1 tablespoon of white vinegar, and 1 tablespoon of lavender essential oil. Mix all the ingredients and keep in an airtight bottle.

◎ Another recipe: in an empty spray bottle, pour 2 tablespoons of shaved *Savon de Marseille*, 1 tablespoon of white vinegar, and 3.4 ounces of hot water. Shake strongly and spray directly on surfaces. Clean and rinse with a sponge.

Refrigerator cleaner

◎ 2 tablespoons of baking soda, the juice of ½ lemon, and 5 drops of lemon essential oil. Dissolve the baking soda in a cup of water. Add the lemon juice and the essential oil. Mix.

Dusting

◎ 1 liter of water, a dot of black soap, and 5 drops of eucalyptus or grapefruit essential oil. Dilute the soap in 1 liter of water. Pour in a spray bottle. Add a few drops of essential oil.

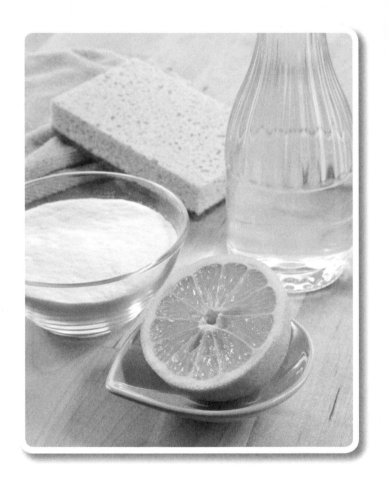

My anti-stress moment

A long period of self-neglect is one of the most probable causes of a panic attack. Take at least one hour per week to "regroup." Here are a few exercises to "harmonize the three levels" of your breath (stomach, lungs, and upper lungs). Relax your abdominals and oxygenate your organs and body.

1. Breathe in at the stomach level. Breathe out slowly. Repeat three times.

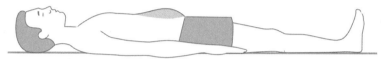

2. Breathe in at the lung level. Breathe out slowly. Repeat three times.

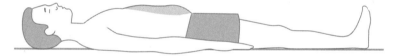

3. Breathe in using your stomach, then the middle and upper lungs, slightly raising your shoulders. Breathe out slowly. Repeat three times.

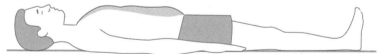

4. Repeat the last three sequences. Add the following each time: soles together, bending your knees to bring your soles toward your perineum.

5. Repeat the last four sequences. Add the following each time: as you inhale, extend your arms above your head. As you exhale, bring them back along your body.

RELAX AND REGULATE YOUR MOODS BEFORE SOMATIZING.

My art therapy moment

✏️ **Your personal dream catcher**

◎ Relax by coloring this dream catcher. Starting in the center, go toward the edges of the page and finish with the feathers.

◎ In a few words, describe the dreams you would like to realize:

. . . .
. . . .
. . . .
. . . .
. . . .
. . . .
. . . .
. . . .
. . . .
. . . .
. . . .
. . . .
. . . .
. . . .
. . . .
. . . .
. . . .
. . . .
. . . .
. . . .

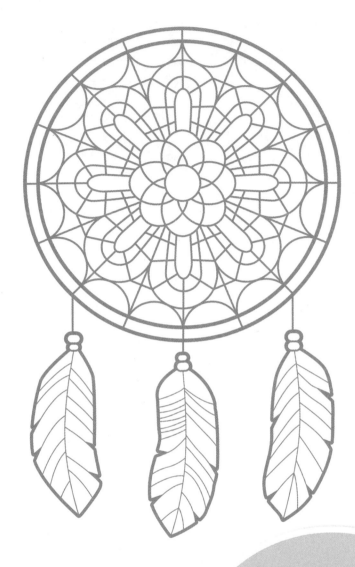

Meditate on this sentence:

He who sees his dream realizes he doesn't need to ever sleep again . . . unless he has other dreams.

Edward D. Wynot

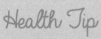

Health Tip

Fists on your torso, breathe in as you open your arms as much as you can; breathe out bringing them together. Breathe in while lifting your arms up; breathe out bringing them back down. Repeat both movements three times.

My path to well-being

The daily maintenance of your body's organs is very simple. These techniques are more preventive than curative, although they can relieve pain.

Intestinal transit

Spread your fingers around your navel. Breathe in while pushing and breathe out while releasing. Repeat for three minutes.

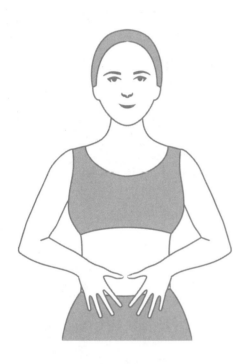

Stomach cramps

Kneeling on the floor, your torso slightly tilted forward, place all your fingertips at the top of your abdomen, under your ribs, and gently push. Breathe while staying in this position for three minutes.

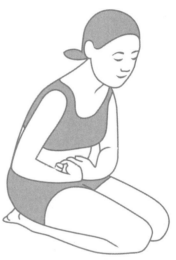

Migraines

Use your right index to gently push above the bridge of your nose, where your right brow starts. Switch sides. Take the time to grab your hair strand by strand, all over your scalp. Finish by massaging your scalp, as if shampooing it.

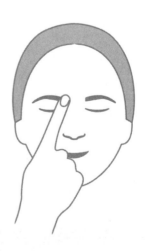

My cocooning space

Acquire a sprouter so you can benefit from the vitamins and minerals of sprouted seeds!

◎   Grains: wheat, barley, oats, spelt, corn, millet, rye, and rice. Also try the seeds of pseudo-grains such as amaranth, buckwheat, and quinoa.

◎   Legumes: alfalfa, red or white beans (but not green), lentils, chickpeas, peas, fenugreek, and mongo beans (or green soya).

◎   Oleaginous: flax, sesame, and sunflower.

◎   Mucilaginous: mustard, watercress, flax, and arugula.

◎   Vegetable: basil, beets, broccoli, carrots, celery, cabbage, fennel, parsley, and radish.

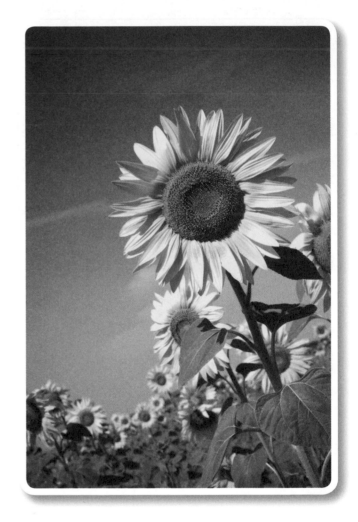

CHEW WELL TO BETTER ABSORB YOUR FOOD'S NUTRITIOUS TREASURES.

My anti-stress moment

Meditating in nature brings pleasure and peace. Here is a productive path to follow at least once a week.

1. Start by walking in a natural environment you like. Let your gaze wander, do not concentrate on anything, and let your eyes roam freely. After a while, stop walking and breathe at your natural rhythm.

2. Close your eyes. Concentrate on far away sounds, then on nearer ones. Now the lower sounds, then the higher pitched ones. Turning to the scents: what does nature smell like? Is it dry or wet? Can you smell the flowers, the sap, the fruits, the decomposing leaves? Do you feel any movement in the air? Let the mood of the place flow in you.

3. Breathe calmly and exhale fully. Rub the palms of your hands together. Then place them on your solar plexus and your stomach, closing your eyes. Using one hand, massage your stomach in clockwise circles while your other hand stays stationary. Rub your hands together again and place them where they were previously: this time, the hand that was on your stomach doesn't move while the other one makes circles on your solar plexus. Stay focused on your breath and let yourself be filled by the energy of the environment without trying to interpret or understand anything. Enjoy the moment . . .

4. Gently rub your face to come back to the moment and resume your activities while trying to prolong this state of well-being.

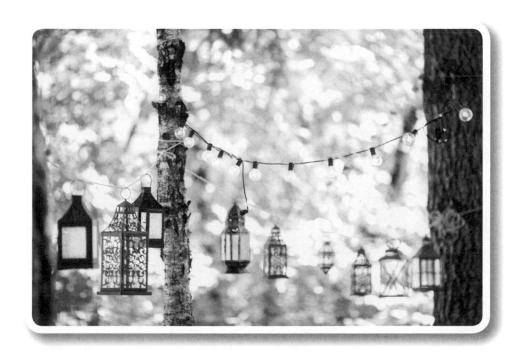

My art therapy moment

✏️ **Multicolor flowers**

◎ Treat yourself to a soft moment by coloring these flowers exclusively with light and soothing colors.

◎ In a few words, describe the softness you perceive in the world around you:

. . . .

. . . .

. . . .

. . . .

. . . .

. . . .

. . . .

. . . .

. . . .

. . . .

. . . .

. . . .

. . . .

. . . .

. . . .

. . . .

Meditate on this sentence:

Beauty originates in the gaze of man. Man's gaze originates in nature.

Hubert Reeves

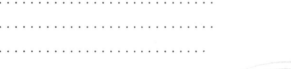

Health Tip

Place the five fingers of your left hand on the left side of your nape; push and release several times, moving your way up towards your scalp. Switch sides.

156

My path to well-being

If you are a cell phone or computer mouse enthusiast, you should know that natural energy doesn't circulate well through your wrists. Here is a path for their daily maintenance. Always respect your feelings and sensations by moving gently.

1. Grab your left wrist with your right hand. Slide the right hand towards the fingers of the left hand that you clench and stretch, all at the same time. Switch hands.

2. Place your palms together, fingers toward the sky, as if in prayer. Raise your elbows keeping your palms together. You are working your forearms and stretching your wrists. Repeat, progressively increasing the number of repetitions.

3. Spread the fingers of your left hand and make a fist with your right hand. Now place your fist between your left fingers, creating a light pressure to stretch each finger. Switch hands.

4. Finish by grabbing your right forearm with your left hand, right below the elbow. Massage by applying pressure and releasing. Repeat all along your forearm. Switch sides.

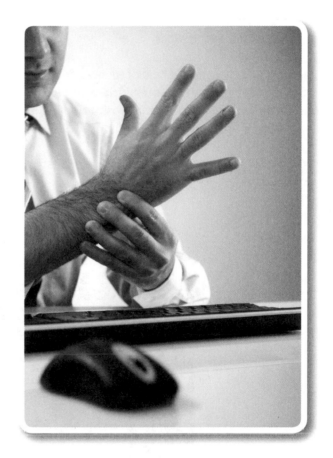

MUSCULOSKELETAL ISSUES NEED CONSTANT CORRECTION.

My cocooning space

A feng shui bedroom is, by definition, a harmonious bedroom. Here are a few basic rules that substantiate why greater simplicity better suits the environment that harbors your sleep, your love, and the regeneration of your body and soul.

◎ You must be able to easily access what you need: closet, chest of drawers, bed, window, lamp, nightstand, etc.

◎ Colors: think soft. Blue and green are associated with serenity and peacefulness. Perfect for a bedroom! You can also use beige, rose, and peach tones.

◎ Sleeping: your bed should be placed away from a window, not opposite a door, and at least ten inches from the floor without anything underneath so that positive energies can circulate freely; if at all possible, orient it north.

◎ Lighting: to create intimacy, choose soft nightstand lamps over ceiling lights.

◎ Interior decoration: stay away from mirrors as they catalyze energy. Avoid cold glass or metal and be sparing with electrical devices: their electromagnetic rays could disturb your sleep.

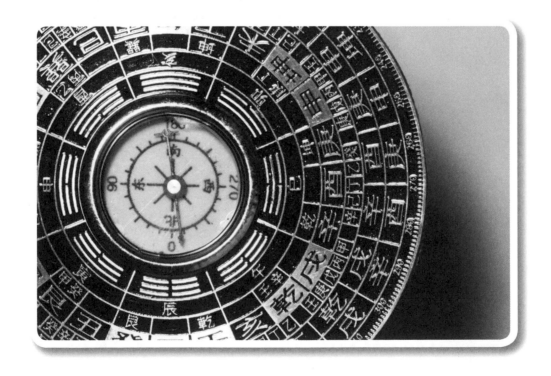

My anti-stress moment

In sophrology, visualization is used to quickly establish a reassuring framework, a positive image of the moment. To construct an image of relaxation by visualization, you first need to accept slow progress, a step-by-step approach. It is essential not to skip any step, not to add any unnecessary element of visualization. This is the only way you will imagine yourself in the mountains before falling asleep, or in a desert in order to concentrate before an important meeting. It is a concrete and practical way to reduce stress. Below is a synopsis that you can adapt and extend depending on your needs.

1. You are lying on a white, sandy beach, breathing slowly. Are you seeing the beach?

2. You are lying on a white, sandy beach and the sky is blue. Are you seeing the blue sky?

3. You are lying on a white, sandy beach, the sky is blue, and a large yellow sun is shining on the horizon. Are you seeing the yellow sun?

4. You are lying on a white, sandy beach, the sky is blue, and a large yellow sun is shining on the horizon. In the ocean there is a boat with beautiful white sails. Are you seeing the boat?

5. You are lying on a white, sandy beach, the sky is blue, and a large yellow sun is shining on the horizon. In the ocean there is a boat with beautiful white sails. A bird offers you to travel on its wings. Do you see the bird?

6. And so on. At each step, add one element. For example: you get on the bird's back and fly over the ocean and meet marvelous friends . . .

7. End your relaxation session by visualizing yourself back on the beach, then into reality, to the here and now.

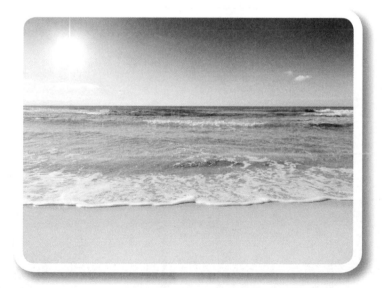

USE YOUR OWN DREAM IMAGES TO BE EVEN MORE ENGAGED.

My art therapy moment

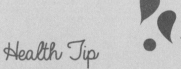

Talk about the people who love you

◎ Starting at the center of this snowflake, use soft and light colors. Work your way to the points using progressively brighter colors.

◎ In a few words, describe people who are close to you and brighten your life:

. . . .
. . . .
. . . .
. . . .
. . . .
. . . .
. . . .
. . . .
. . . .
. . . .
. . . .
. . . .
. . . .
. . . .
. . . .
. . . .
. . . .
. . . .
. . . .

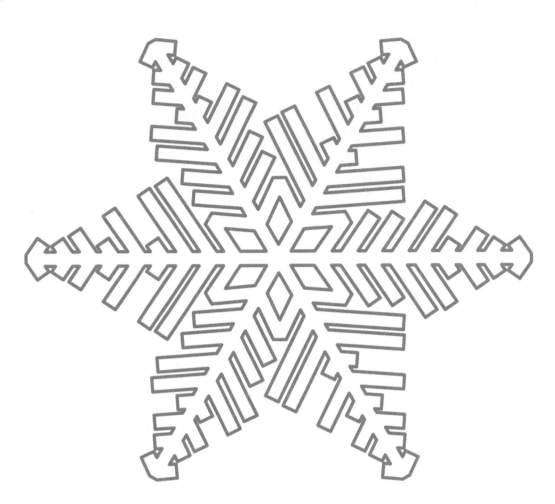

Meditate on this sentence:

Each flower is a soul that blossoms in nature.

Gérard de Nerval

Health Tip

Light a soft-colored candle (pastel green or blue) to accompany you during your peaceful art therapy sessions.

160

My path to well-being

You can practice yoga discreetly and gently at the office. It is an excellent tool to maintain your form and to avoid accumulating stress.

1. Sitting on the edge of a chair, back straight, inhale and exhale while turning your head to the left. Come back to your original position, then turn your head right. Come back to your original position. Inhale while stretching your head up; exhale while bringing it down.

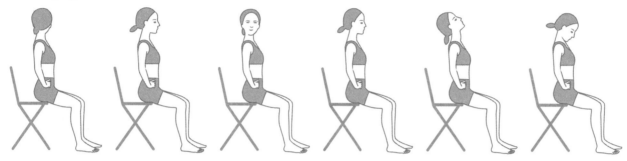

2. Still on the edge of a chair, inhale while extending your left arm toward the floor and extending your right arm toward the ceiling. Switch sides. Repeat at least three times.

3. On the edge of your chair, place your fists on your abdomen, above your navel; lean forward so you can exhale all the air from your lungs and come back up. Repeat three times.

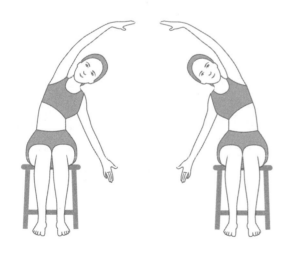

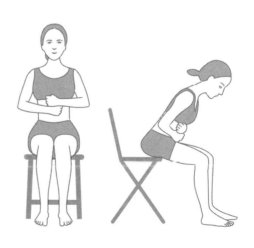

PRACTICE EASY REMEDIAL POSTURE POSES, EVEN AT THE OFFICE.

My cocooning space

 Most of the time, our feet are confined in shoes. Worse, although our feet bear the weight of our body and provide balance and stability, we rarely pay attention to them. Below are a few ideas for their care!

Dry feet

◎ **Recipe 1:** Mix 2 tablespoons of fine salt with 2 tablespoons of olive or argan oil. Massage your feet with this mixture, particularly the heels. Rinse and let your feet soak in lukewarm, lemony water. Dry them and massage with a few drops of argan oil for guaranteed softness.

◎ **Recipe 2:** Mix the juice of ½ a lemon, 1 tablespoon of almond oil, and 2 tablespoons of coarse or fine salt. Massage your feet using circular movements. Rinse, dry, and apply your usual foot hydrating cream.

Tired feet

◎ Dilute ½ glass of baking soda in a kitchen basin of lukewarm water. Let your feet soak 15 minutes.

Nail care

◎ To treat and strengthen your toe nails, massage them with lukewarm olive oil. For in-depth cleaning, regularly rub your toenails with ½ lemon.

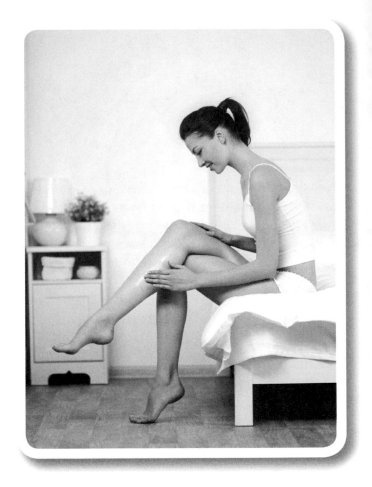

Group exchange

Many people around you have extraordinary tales to tell! People's stories are full of anecdotes and knowledge that beg to be conveyed. The idea is to collect these stories and share them on an association or group site.

Stories to share

◎ On the occasion of a community celebration, set up a stand or share one with an existing municipal or regional organization.

◎ Prepare flyers explaining the objective of your project. Get organized so an original biography (electronic or paper) comes out every month: the story of a traditional trade told by its last practitioner; memories of somebody who has a deep knowledge of the town and its history, etc.

◎ When they actually see the concrete results of your partnership, people will be more inclined to talk.

Information to share

◎ Offer to meet with an author and tape a story before its publication. Think about asking for a written permission before disseminating the text (agreement without monetary exchange).

◎ You are in fact creating a fascinating historical record of your town. After that, you are ready to enrich the adventure to larger or more specialized topics.

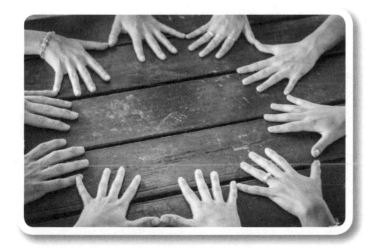

LOCAL HISTORY UNIFIES AND INVITES PEOPLE TO OPEN UP.

Group creativity

Creative recycling is a very simple way to utilize objects people have discarded, either by raffling them off or selling them within the framework of an organization. The operating words are: collect, valorize, sell, and raise awareness.

1. Define your project: for example, personalize old toys or pieces of furniture. Organize a team of creative people who will refurbish, strip, paint them, etc.

2. Collect: teaming up with the local authority, find a drop-off space. Think about specifying the type of objects you accept (furniture and toys, for example!)

3. Valorize: this is where creativity becomes essential. Each member of the team brings his or her specific know-how to the project. If you get damaged but original chairs, name a project manager who will establish a step-by-step valorization plan: strip, paint, add decorative elements, etc. Each member's experience is welcome, under the supervision of the project manager. Use the same process for toys. Hear out everyone's ideas and appoint a project manager to orchestrate them. This is a proven and effective organizational structure!

4. Sell or exchange: yard sales, flea markets, rummage and barter sales, every event is an opportunity to sell or exchange while publicizing the principle of mutualityand reinvest in a larger network!

5. Raise awareness: create a site or small signs to explain how every one can recycle discarded objects and propose an alternative approach to consumerism. The idea is to progress, starting from a selective choice to productive recycling.

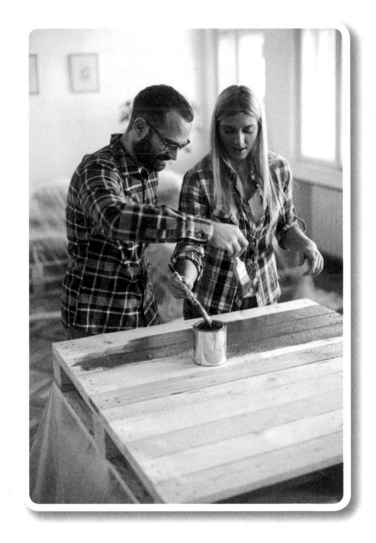

Art therapy collective

When used in a group, there are many benefits to music therapy. Try physically reacting to rhythms, then coloring pictures to express feelings. A complete creative path! To organize a collective music therapy session you will need a performance space, white sheets of paper, and coloring pens. To remain coherent, try to organize small groups of five or less.

1. The group gathers around the activity organizer, who explains the session. This can also be done by e-mail if the participants already know one another. Each person has to bring three types of music, chosen according to the following criteria:

◎ A very rhythmic piece that induces tension release (for some, it will be Mozart; for others, Metallica. No judgment!)

◎ A piece of relaxing music. It might go from lounge music or jazz to rock or classical music. There is no right or wrong!

◎ A piece of soft but dynamic music. Happy, suggestive, lively, such as tropical music, bossa nova, etc.

2. Each piece is about fifteen minutes long. The leader choses four pieces for their cohesion. If every one feels up to it, there might be two sessions of four fifteen-minute pieces, for a total of two hours.

3. While listening, participants let their bodies express their feelings by dancing, sitting, drawing, or reclining. Between musical pieces participants are encouraged to verbalize, without being judged. The group can be given a ten-minute coloring break, either free-form or on a collectively chosen topic.

4. At the end of the session participants thank each other. It is advisable to choose another leader for the next session.

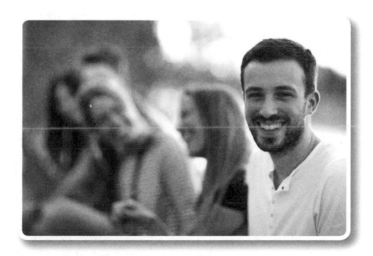

MUSIC AND RHYTHM HARMONIZE A GROUP.

Assess your stress regularly. It only takes a few minutes! Add a massage and, voilà: inner harmony is restored in no time.

1. Breathe gently; then, starting from the top to the bottom of your body, like a scanner, feel whether your face is tense. If so, inhale and exhale, charging your breath with a well-being feeling and mentally sending it to the sensitive points. Do not hesitate to add a massage as you check yourself—forehead, temples, ears, etc.

2. Continue down to your torso, your hips, and your legs. Massage to relax, if only for a few minutes. Each time, send your body a positive thought. Your breath accompanies this constructive act. You are taking care of yourself, taking care of your body, this earthly vehicle. In this life, you only have this one body. Be gentle with it. Love it! Being attentive to your health and your well-being is an essential meditation.

3. Take a few minutes to scribble on a piece of paper. Let your mind relax. Express your thoughts, your nervousness, in rapid or slow strokes on a white sheet. Write words, or letters, or use the tip of your pen for dots. Unwind . . .

4. When you feel calmer, take a few appeasing breaths, i.e. exhale longer than you inhale. Come back and concentrate on yourself, feel your inner peace, check your body posture, rectify it if necessary (back straight but not tense, etc.) Finally, crumple or tear the piece of paper, throwing it in a wastebasket with the firm intention of moving on.

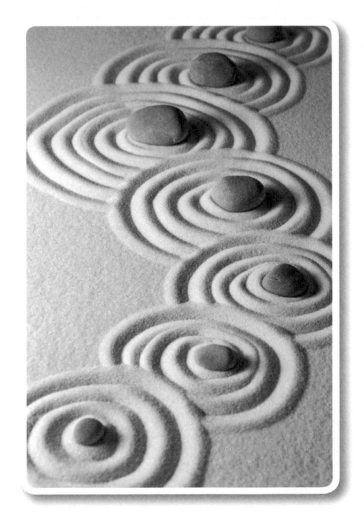

My art therapy moment

✏ Decide to act

◎ Here is a multi-shape expression mandala. Start by coloring the central circle with bright colors, then venture outward to the larger circle with light colors and the triangle with the colors of your choice.

◎ In a few words, synthetize the decisions that you plan on making in order to improve your quality of life:

....

....

....

....

....

....

....

....

....

....

....

....

....

....

....

....

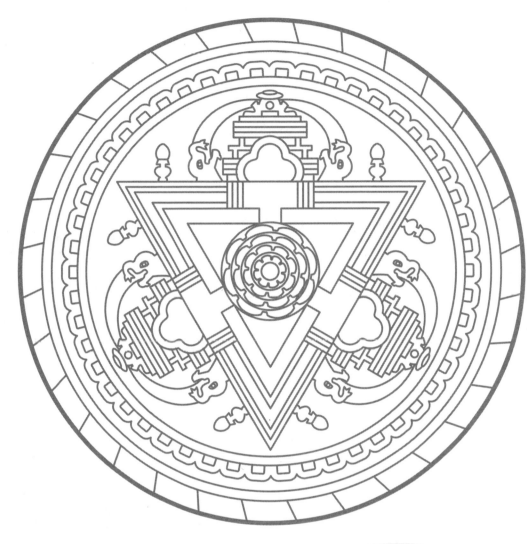

Meditate on this sentence:

I wish I could, if only once, really decide to be healthy!

Georg Christoph Lichtenberg

Health Tip

Take time to regularly concentrate on this type of mandala; it will bring relaxation and mental peace.

My path to well-being

Our eyes can use up to 80 percent of our body's energy to function properly. Work the visual system with well-focused exercises that prevent mental fatigue and migraines.

◎ Sitting on a chair, head straight, feet flat on the floor, hands on your knees, move your eyes from left to right without moving your head. Repeat ten times rather quickly while breathing calmly.

◎ Without moving your head, look toward the floor. Inhale as your eyes look up to the ceiling; exhale as your eyes go down vertically to the ground. Repeat about ten times, slowly, while breathing naturally.

◎ Imagine a point in front of you within your visual field. Move your eyes horizontally and go in large circles around the point five times clockwise, five times counterclockwise, while breathing calmly. Still going in large circles from the central point, move your eyes upward then to the right, returning to the top before getting back to your original position.

◎ Make a large X: your eyes go obliquely bottom right to top left; horizontally to top left; top left to bottom right. Reverse top left to bottom right; horizontally to bottom left to top right.

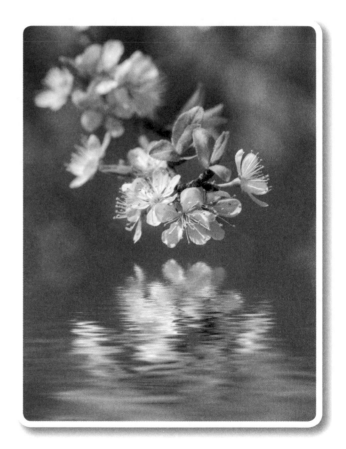

VISION BALANCE IS PRIMORDIAL TO LIVE STRESS-FREE!

My cocooning space

 Eyes are sensitive: take care of them, your face in general, and the area around the eyes in particular. You will look rested and protect yourself from the oxidant effects of pollution.

Make-up remover

You need: 1.7 ounces of macadamia oil, 0.7 ounces of castor oil, 0.7 ounces of aloe vera, and 0.7 ounces of cornflower hydrolat (floral water).

◎ Sterilize a 1.7 ounce plastic jar, preferably opaque so light does not affect the ingredient properties. Using a funnel, put the macadamia and castor oils in the jar. Add the aloe vera and the cornflower hydrolat. Shake the jar before using.

◎ Dab some make-up removing lotion on a wet cotton round. Apply to your eyelids and eyelashes for a few minutes. Then, rub it back and forth a few times on your eyelids. Repeat several times if necessary.

Homemade Honey Exfoliation

You need: 1 tablespoon of liquid honey, 1 teaspoon of almond powder, 1 teaspoon of powdered sugar, and a few drops of orange blossom water.

◎ Clean your face with soap and water. Dry.

◎ Mix the ingredients in a bowl. Apply on your face, avoiding the area around the eyes and the eyelids. Keep on for 2 minutes.

◎ With the tip of your fingers, gently massage your face.

◎ Rinse with lukewarm water. Use tonic water and a good hydrating cream suitable to your skin type.

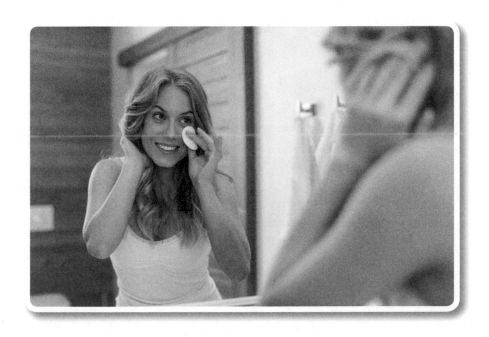

My anti-stress moment

Focused meditation is an intense process that uses the power of concentration. It is progressive. You start with a precise concentration point to which elements are added step-by-step. You go beyond your stress and quickly obtain inner harmony. Keep in mind that stress occurs as a normal reaction of your body to an outer stimulus (an aggressive person, a difficult situation, etc.) or to an inner stimulus (irritability, personal anger). As the creator of your stress, you can take action to diminish it!

1. Start with choosing a point of attention: a pragmatic object that does not induce distraction, like the picture of your child. Choose a non-stimulating object—some people use a car key to avoid slipping into day dreaming. Look at the object for three minutes; this should slow down your breathing. If a thought comes to you, focus your attention back on the object, its shape, its color. Your attention is only riveted on this object!

2. Your eyes still on your point of attention, take three minutes to concentrate on sounds. Nothing else is of interest to you but wood creaking, cars, birds, people in the street. . . . If your mind digresses toward a feeling, like "hunger" for example, concentrate back on your point of attention and sounds.

3. Your eyes still concentrated on the object and your ears on the sounds, take another three minutes to acknowledge how your body feels: slumping shoulders need straightening up, arm muscles are a little tense, your face, etc. Progress in your meditation practice by adding more and more points of attention.

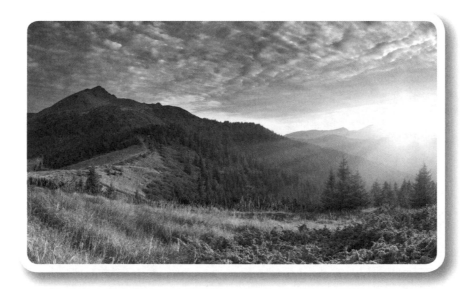

MEDITATION DEVELOPS CONCENTRATION.

My art therapy moment

✏️ Take time to concentrate some more

◎ Start by using yellow in the center. Progress towards the exterior, finishing each concentric portion of the mandala before starting another one. With the yellow in the center as an anchor, produce a harmonious drawing by using soft and vivacious colors.

◎ List a few words that symbolize concentration for you:

. . . .

. . . .

. . . .

. . . .

. . . .

. . . .

. . . .

. . . .

. . . .

. . . .

. . . .

. . . .

. . . .

Meditate on this sentence:

Calm is a creative element. It concentrates, purifies, organizes inner forces.

Stefan Zweig

Health Tip

To clarify your ideas, massage the center of your forehead with the tip of your index finger for one minute.

My well-being path

Here are two maps to inconspicuously massage a few essential hand reflexology points in order to relax, whenever and wherever: at work, during your commute, or at home watching a good movie. The method is simple: place your thumb on a reflexology point and, without causing pain, gently drill it in and release it several times. Do not worry. Take care of yourself!

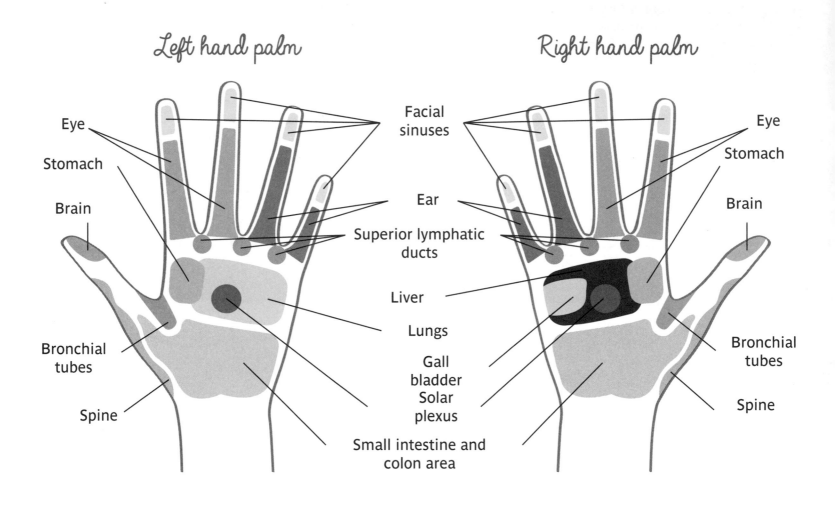

Left hand palm

Right hand palm

Eye
Stomach
Brain
Bronchial tubes
Spine

Facial sinuses
Ear
Superior lymphatic ducts
Liver
Lungs
Gall bladder
Solar plexus
Small intestine and colon area

Eye
Stomach
Brain
Bronchial tubes
Spine

◎ Always work several points together. For example, to encourage digestion, massage the liver, gallbladder, intestine, and stomach points. Massage the sinuses and eye points to balance your vision.

◎ Regularly massage the zone corresponding to your solar plexus to balance your moods.

REFLEXOLOGY IS A POWERFUL, HEALTH-ENHANCING TOOL.

My cocooning space

In antiquity, magnetic forces were frequently used in medical treatments. The technique is based on the fact that certain ailments are due to a temporary magnetic field imbalance that affects the functioning of the body. The best therapeutic magnets are the neodymium magnets, also called "rare earth" magnets. The contact of these magnets with the affected or painful area accelerates blood circulation, spreading the magnetic field further into the body and interrupting the transmission of the pain signal between the organ and the brain.

◎ Magnets relieve inflammation and, more particularly, muscular and articular pains (arthritis, arthrosis, rheumatisms . . .)
as well as migraines and back pains. They are useful to prevent traumatic edema.

◎ Since they rebalance energy, magnets are occasionally used for sleep disorders. We strongly recommend seeking medical advice, ideally in a sports medicine center because many athletes use magnets to avoid taking anti-inflammatory drugs.

◎ Magnets are available in knee and elbow pads, lumbar belts (extended sitting positions or carrying heavy loads) or as individual pieces to be inserted in appropriate harnesses.

◎ Magnets last a lifetime. They are easy to use, affordable, and can be shared by the whole family. An excellent investment!

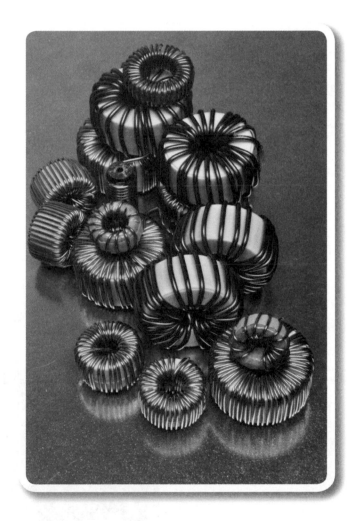

My anti-stress moment

Focalized Meditation (see last week) can be practiced alone, as a family, or at work. Also called mindful meditation, it fosters a realistic perception of life, taking things one moment at a time, without letting the mind create imaginary circumstances or emotions construct inappropriate behaviors.

◎ At the beginning, it is best to plan your meditation sessions. Use some of your less tense moments at work to focus on an object for one minute and to slow down your breathing.

◎ Once in harmony, forget about the world around you. Focus on what is and what is happening, while concentrating on your point of attention.

◎ Your colleagues walk by your desk, but you simply observe somebody walking by, without giving in to interpretation: instead of "my colleague is walking by quickly, she must be stressed," stop at "a colleague is walking by."

◎ Your eyes still concentrated on the object, you hear noises. Take mental note of the noise. It only enters your present. If your mind starts interjecting ("oh, this is a bus and there are people in the street") come back to your object of attention.

◎ If you are able to do this regularly, at least once in the morning and once in the afternoon, you will relax deeply in no time. 70 percent of our stress comes from the pressure created by our mind or our emotions. De-stressing depends on regular practice!

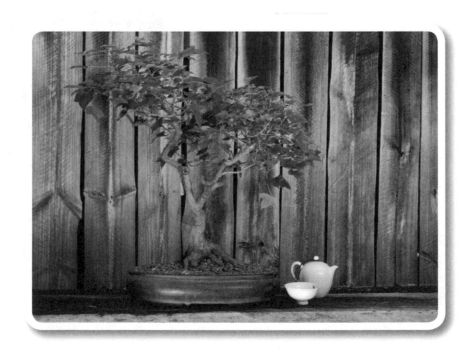

My art-therapy moment

✏️ **Talk about your travel fantasies**

◎ Start from the outside border, coloring each element clockwise, if possible. Change colors every time!

◎ List a few words that evoke escape and travel:

....

....

....

....

....

....

....

....

....

....

....

....

....

....

....

....

....

....

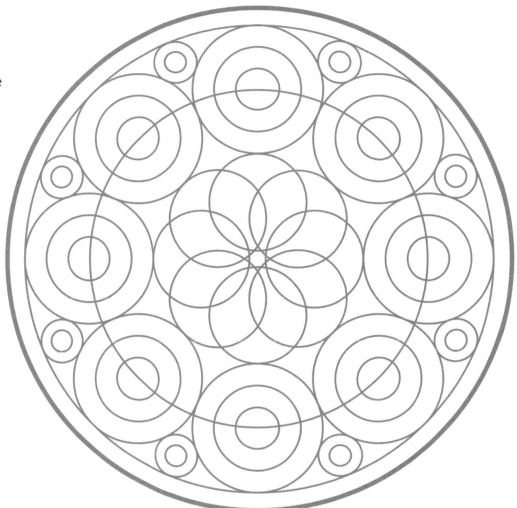

Meditate on this sentence:

To stay put is to exist. To travel is to live.

Gustave Nadaud

Health Tip

Several times a day, let your eye wander on something green, for peace; then on something yellow, for concentration.

My path to well-being

After learning to massage our hands, let us learn to massage our feet reflexology points! Our feet provide support to our body and align our hips and spine. For an even deeper relaxation, complement the massage with a salt-water footbath.

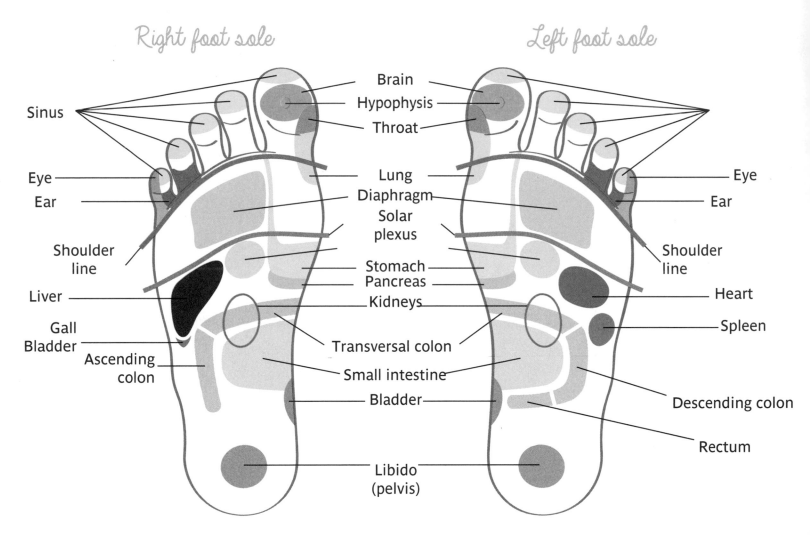

Right foot sole

Left foot sole

Brain
Hypophysis
Throat

Sinus

Eye
Ear

Shoulder line

Liver

Gall Bladder

Ascending colon

Lung
Diaphragm
Solar plexus

Stomach
Pancreas
Kidneys

Transversal colon

Small intestine

Bladder

Libido (pelvis)

Eye
Ear

Shoulder line

Heart

Spleen

Descending colon

Rectum

◎ Start by massaging your heels. They bear much of our body weight and adapt in order to balance our body. They need to be treated gently.

◎ Using your hands, identify all the painful reflexology points. Take time to relax them; then check the organ to which they correspond.

◎ Always end by stretching your toes and wriggling them around gently.

BODY STRETCHES REBOOT THE NERVOUS SYSTEM.

My cocooning space

Natural light is necessary for our organism to fight stress and sudden slumps. Light therapy has become more and more common, above all in the winter and in places where natural light is rare or nonexistent.

◎ Light intensity is expressed in lux. In the summer, we are exposed to 10,000 lux. A basic home light provides 50 to 100 lux. Make sure to check how many lux your device produces: the higher the number of lux, the lower the exposure time. For example, it takes two hours to recharge with a 2,500-lux device but less than thirty minutes with a 10,000 lux.

◎ The recommended distance is twelve feet for a 10,000 lux. To better absorb the light through your retina, keep your eyes open and place the lamp right above your normal gaze line.

◎ You can read or write while using your light therapy lamp. Place it opposite you without looking at the bulb directly. If you choose a low lux lamp, bring it closer; it will be just as efficient as a high intensity lamp placed further.

◎ Note that it is essential to use your lamp consistently. Effects will be noticeable after four to five days. Daily usage is recommended from October 15 to March 31. If you work nights or get off work late in the day, do not hesitate to use a light therapy lamp year-round to make up the energy loss.

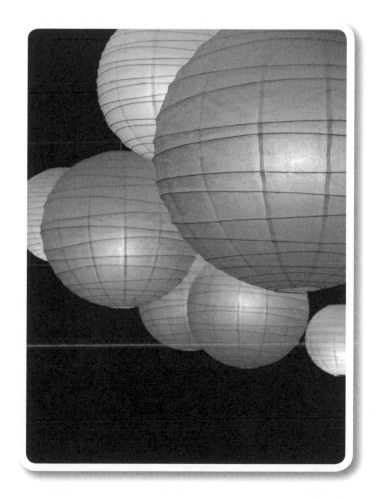

My anti-stress moment

Most people think it's normal to experience tension every day. A day at work creates tensions, right? The objective of the meditation session offered here is to break the constant stress you are used to dealing with every day. You will become present to every moment of your life, as if someone had pinched you! You can practice this anywhere, anytime.

◎   For one hour, you decide to take some distance. It does not mean that you retreat from life. You consciously listen and observe life. For example, you take a few minutes before you engage in a verbal response, you wait a bit before your body starts moving, you breathe deeply three times before making a phone call, etc., just enough to breakout of the usual cycle of events, which are quite often out of our control.

◎   Day after day, this small distance will prevent you from expending your energy as if it were a bottomless tank whose gauge you do not need to check. It will make you aware of stress alerts and force you to take them into account!

◎   Once every hour, standing or sitting, stop for a short moment. Listen and look, become aware of what is happening around you. By doing so, you are putting meaning back in your activities. After you reaffirm your desire to be part of these activities, re-engage in your present.

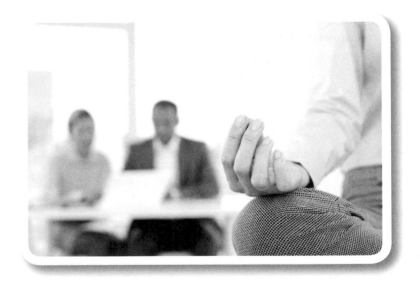

DE-STRESS BY PUTTING MEANING BACK IN YOUR DAY.

My art therapy moment

Simply reassess

◎ This mandala must represent you. In the central circle, use a color that represents you today. In the four smaller circles, enter the emotional states that characterize you best (joy, anxiety, etc.). Enter one in each circle, adding more circles on the exterior row of the mandala if needed. Use the color that suits each emotion best.

◎ In a few words, describe the origin of these feelings (actions, education, duty):

. . . .
. . . .
. . . .
. . . .
. . . .
. . . .
. . . .
. . . .
. . . .
. . . .
. . . .
. . . .
. . . .
. . . .
. . . .

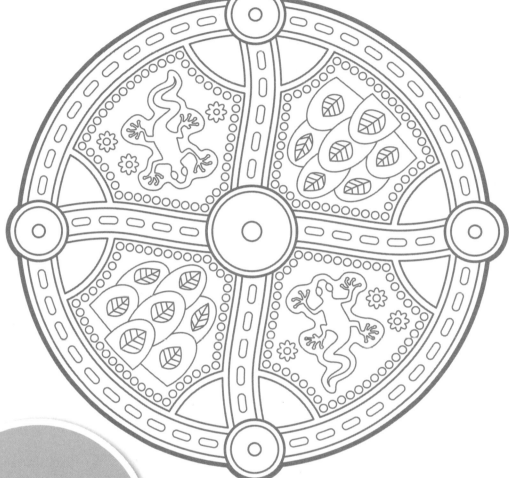

Meditate on this sentence:

To love is to take a trip to the edges of yourself.

Hélène Ouvrard

Coaching Tip

Take inconspicuous breaks: elbows on your desk, place the tips of your fingers together. Push and release a few times to relax.

My path to well-being

Conscious energy work is a necessary phase of de-stressing. Here we offer a very simple approach to consciously maintaining your chakras, also called wheel of strength or wheel of light in the West. You will be able to familiarize yourself with the seven main chakras and learn to act on them once a week.

1. The primary objective is to reach inner peace. Start rubbing the palms of your hands together to warm them up. Place one hand on the heart chakra, in the middle of your torso. Pull your hand away a few inches then put it back on your torso. Repeat as if your palm were a suction cup that reinforces your heart's energy

2. Use this very simple movement on the seven chakras of your body, as indicated on the drawing below. Breathe very calmly.

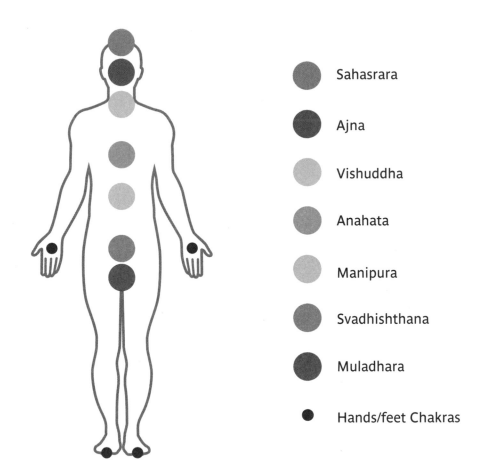

- Sahasrara
- Ajna
- Vishuddha
- Anahata
- Manipura
- Svadhishthana
- Muladhara
- Hands/feet Chakras

ALWAYS BE MINDFUL OF YOUR PERSONAL ENERGY LEVEL.

My cocooning space

Grains dubbed "ancient" are popular again because they are easier to digest. With allergies and food intolerances on the rise (gluten, sub-par quality starches, etc.), consumers are resorting to grains to break free from quotas or extensive agriculture. Below are a few examples.

Small spelt or Einkorn

◎ This grain dates back to 9000 BC and has never been modified!

◎ It does not require pesticides and is the only germinate that contains all the amino acids essential to humans.

◎ Moreover, 3.4 ounces of small spelt provides 0.3 ounces of fiber, which increases the feeling of satiety while being hypoallergenic.

Millet

◎ Originally from Asia and Africa, this hypoallergenic grain is rich in vitamin A and contains rare minerals such as manganese and zinc.

Barley

◎ Very rich in fiber, it is beneficial to the digestive process. Used both as a main course and a pastry ingredient (it is very sweet!).

◎ Not only does it make you feel full, it also boasts glycaemia regulatory properties and lowers cholesterol.

Corn

◎ Rich in protein, iron, calcium, and fiber, corn is easy to cook and pleases the whole family.

◎ There are many varieties around the world and it is consumed in different forms (semolina, grains, flakes, patties, etc.).

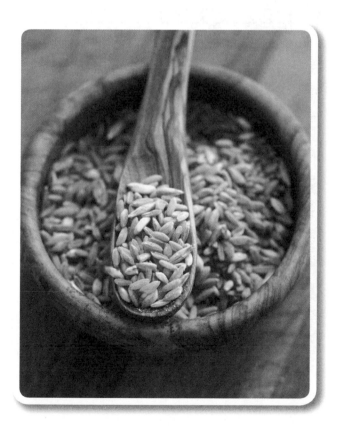

My anti-stress moment

Breathing can very quickly bring you peace. The more attentive you are to your breathing, the more consciously you will be able to use it in key moments of your life, curatively or even preventively, when you know that you are going to be exposed to a stressful situation. A few breaths should be enough to instantly restore peace.

Movement

◎ Close your eyes and extend your arms out horizontally while breathing in through the nose. Imagine that the air is flowing in through both your palms, moving along your arms, into your whole body, and filling your lungs.

◎ Slowly breathe out through your lips while you cross your arms on your chest. Imagine the air leaving your body not only through your mouth but also through the top of your head and the soles of your feet.

◎ This breathing sequence is called "the cross" because, symbolically, breathing in is done horizontally while breathing out is done vertically. Repeat at least seven times.

Visualization

◎ Slowly breathe in through the nose, imagining that the air is circulating through your stomach then coming back up along your back to arrive to your head.

◎ Breathe out, through the nose, if possible. The air leaves your body but its strength continues to travel through your face, your neck, and the middle of your torso to stop right under your navel.

◎ Repeat seven times.

Touch

◎ Right palm in your left palm, breathe in, placing both your palms under your navel, then in the middle of your torso, and in the middle of your forehead.

◎ Breathe out while bringing your palms under your navel. Repeat seven times.

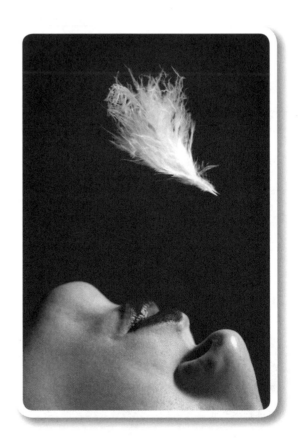

ADD A THOUGHT OF PERSONAL LOVE AND RESPECT TO YOUR BREATHING.

My art therapy moment

 Represent your tenderness

◎ Softly color these sweet leaves yellow and green. Take some time to breathe, feel calm. Finish by drawing flowers to color pink and white.

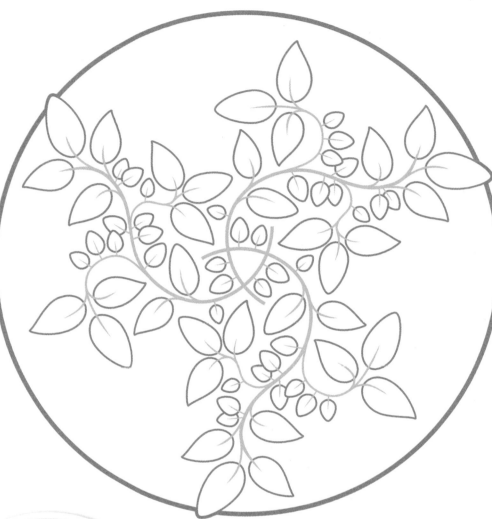

◎ Write a few words about poetry and tenderness:

. . . .

. . . .

. . . .

. . . .

. . . .

. . . .

. . . .

. . . .

. . . .

. . . .

. . . .

. . . .

. . . .

Meditate on this sentence:

Without dream, poetry is impossible. Without poetry, life is intolerable.

Louis Pasteur Vallery-Radot

Health Tip

Remember to drink water regularly: it is necessary for our body to function properly, digest nutrients, and eliminate toxins.

My path to well-being

Qigong encourages concentration, augments lung capacity, and promotes listening to your body, all in silence. Here is a first series of movements. While doing these, concentrate on feeling the exercise and on breathing regularly.

1. Breathe in, palms open toward the ceiling. Raise your arms up to your nose. Turn your palms in and bring up your arms while slowly breathing out. Repeat seven times.

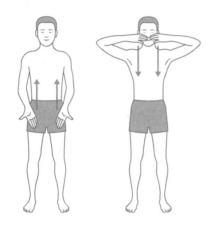

3. Arms resting along your body, inhale while bringing your slightly bent arms up, palms turned toward the floor. Exhale, bringing your arms back along your body. Repeat seven times.

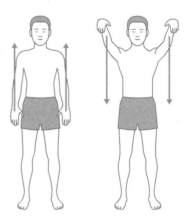

2. Turn your torso to the right while exhaling, lifting your left hand to the right and your right hand to the left. Breathe in and switch sides. Repeat three times.

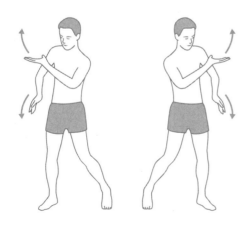

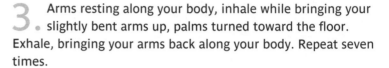

SLOWER MOVEMENTS ARE MORE EFFICIENT.

My cocooning space

A good source of fiber, puréed vegetables are real treasures, if you are willing to innovate a little. Light in texture, they are ideal for an evening meal, as they do not overtax your intestines during the night's digestion process.

Fresh green peas and shallots purée

You will need: 3 to 3.5 pounds of fresh green peas, 6.7 to 7 ounces heavy cream, 12 green shallots, salt, and pepper.

◎ Cook the shelled fresh green peas in boiling water for 12 minutes.

◎ Drain and cut them to purée them in a blender with the heavy cream. Add salt and pepper.

◎ Cut the green shallots and add them to the purée, serve piping hot!

Watercress purée

You will need: 4 bunches of watercress, 3 ounces of butter, freshly grated nutmeg, salt, and pepper.

◎ Clean the watercress, discarding the hard stems. Cut them coarsely.

◎ Place in cold, salted water. Bring to a boil and leave 1 minute, no more. Drain well before pureeing in a blender.

◎ Melt the butter in a pan; add the watercress and mix to homogenize. Add nutmeg, salt, and pepper to taste. Serve hot!

Fennel purée

You will need: 1 garlic clove, 4 fennel bulbs, 2 lemons, salt, pepper, and a sprinkling of olive oil.

◎ Preheat the oven at 320 degrees F. Wrap the garlic in aluminum foil. Cook in the oven for 30 minutes.

◎ Boil 1 liter of water. Wash the 4 fennel bulbs. Zest and juice the lemons. Place the fennel in the boiling water with the lemon juice and zests. Allow to simmer 20 to 25 minutes.

◎ Drain the fennels and purée with the peeled garlic cloves. Add a sprinkling of olive oil and season to taste right before serving.

Eggplant purée

You will need: 6 eggplants, 1 garlic clove, ½ lemon, 1 tablespoon of sesame oil, 1 tablespoon of olive oil, salt, and pepper.

◎ Preheat the oven at 350 degrees F. Cut the eggplants lengthwise, wrap them in aluminum foil, and bake them for 45 minutes.

◎ When they are ready, take the meat out of the skins and reserve. Discard the skins.

◎ Add the crushed garlic and the juice of ½ lemon to the eggplants. Incorporate 1 tablespoon of sesame oil and 1 tablespoon of olive oil.

◎ Warm all the ingredients in a pot. Adjust seasoning to taste and serve.

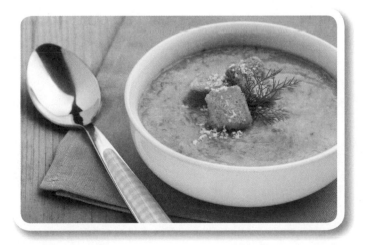

Relaxing can be very quick if you subtly succeed in severing your dependency on stress. Compassion for somebody else is one method to succeed! Unmanaged stress is very invasive. Concentrating on a strong and diverting feeling will give you a sufficient impulsion to distance yourself from your own stress. At first, it is more efficient to link movement and feeling, which will reinforce your will to transition from stress to giving. Practice this regularly to establish a reflex.

◎   As soon as you feel stressed, take a moment to breathe calmly and turn towards somebody you trust. If there is nobody around, think about somebody in particular. Put your right hand on your heart and send a real feeling of love: breathe in while taking a little piece of your heart, breathe out sending the feeling out to the person. Repeat several times and calmly breathe again.

◎   If you have time and space to do so, join your right and left hands, opened toward the ceiling, and place them a few inches away from your stomach. While inhaling, lift up your palms at the level of your throat, imagining they are receiving all your feelings, your love, your wish to give. . . . Exhale while opening your arms to offer your realization wishes to the whole world.

◎   In this precise moment, you interrupt what you were thinking or doing to send a positive thought to somebody. If it is simpler, think it intently as you continue your daily activities, but keep the thought in your mind for two to three minutes as a mantra with the intention that the positive energy brings well-being to the person you have in mind.

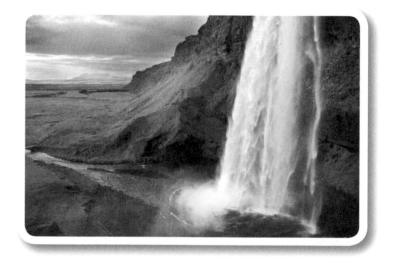

COMPASSION OPENS THE HEART AND RESCUES IT FROM STRESS.

My art therapy moment

✏️ Words of love for somebody else

◎ Color all these hearts at your own rhythm, associating a person to whom you wish to bring comfort.

◎ Write a few words of love:

. . . .

. . . .

. . . .

. . . .

. . . .

. . . .

. . . .

. . . .

. . . .

. . . .

. . . .

. . . .

. . . .

. . . .

. . . .

. . . .

. . . .

Meditate on this sentence:

Love is the only thing that keeps one alive.

Oscar Wilde

Coaching Tip

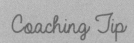

As soon as it feels itchy, massage your throat with ravensara essential oil. It will get better in no time.

My path to well-being

1. Your arms above your head, slowly move your upper body to the right, then to the left. Repeat for two minutes, slowly.

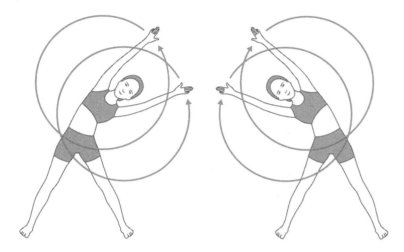

2. Your right palm towards the floor, inhale as you raise your right palm and your left foot. Switch sides. Repeat for two minutes.

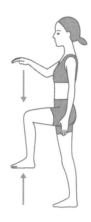

3. Arms along your body, put your weight on your left leg while bringing your left arm up. Slowly extend your right foot so only your big toe touches the floor. Round your left arm above your head stretching your left side. Use your right arm for balance. Repeat for two minutes and switch sides.

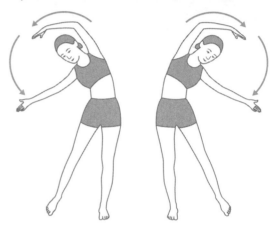

4. Standing up, arms along your body, inhale as you extend your arms above your head. Exhale as you bend your torso at a forty-five degree angle and bring your arms down to your knees. Repeat seven times.

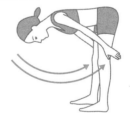

My cocooning space

 Learn not to waste food.

Orange peel

◎ Contrary to popular belief, orange peel is good for our health! It protects our body from inflammation and heart disease, so do not hesitate to add some zest to your dishes (after washing the peel).

Apple peel

◎ Apple peel contains more vitamins and fiber than the flesh of the fruit. Its antioxidants (quercitrin) are beneficial to our lungs and brain.

◎ Choose organic apples and wash them before eating their skin.

Potato skin (thoroughly cleaned)

◎ Potato skins contain vitamins B and C, calcium, potassium, and iron. Choose organic potatoes so you can bake them with their skin!

Beet greens

◎ Beet greens contain vitamins and calcium. Serve as salad or cooked, like spinach!

Turnip greens

◎ Full of iron, magnesium, vitamins, and fiber, turnip greens are excellent for our health. Cook them at the same time as the turnips themselves.

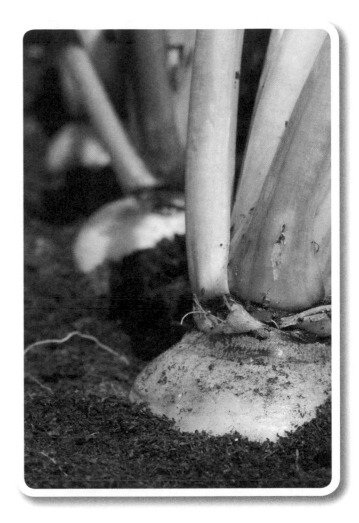

WE MUST LEARN TO BECOME MINDFUL CONSUMERS.

My anti-stress moment

Cardiac coherence requires you to be mindful of your breathing rhythm, then to impose a rhythm of six breathing cycles (inhale, exhale) per minute. This is the cardiac rhythm at which your nervous system and your cells function harmoniously.

◎ Researchers offer the following count, instituted progressively: a five-second inhale and a five-second exhale repeated over five-minute phases, once in the morning and once in the afternoon. Of course, you might need a natural respiratory pause between inhale and exhale. First and foremost, listen to your body. Practiced regularly, these will be quite beneficial! Simply remember to sit down with your back straight. You might want to place your right index finger on the inside of your wrist to monitor your pulse and its evolution: physically registering the appeasement is quite a constructive notion!

◎ Once this meditation is well established, you will associate four types of positive sentences that you will express with determination so they expand a powerful creative energy. For example:

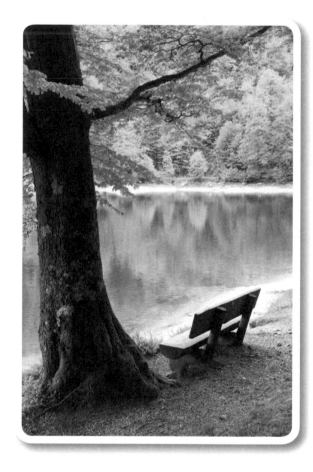

  ◎ A personal sentence: "I am in good health."

  ◎ A personal commitment sentence: "I am setting up a glowing future."

  ◎ A collective wish sentence: "I commit to bring harmony around me."

  ◎ A compassion sentence: "I bring attention to my unhappy cousin."

CARDIAC COHERENCE IS EFFICIENT AND SUPER SIMPLE.

My art therapy moment

✏️ **Available to oneself**

◎ Reach your cardiac coherence and use a different color for each part of the mandala, without paying attention to the possible thoughts that might break your concentration.

◎ Write a few words on the idea of linkage to one's own source:

. . . .
. . . .
. . . .
. . . .
. . . .
. . . .
. . . .
. . . .
. . . .
. . . .
. . . .
. . . .
. . . .
. . . .
. . . .
. . . .
. . . .
. . . .
. . . .
. . . .
. . . .

Meditate on this sentence:

Happiness is not found, it is made. Happiness doesn't depend on what we don't have but on how we use what we have.

Arnaud Desjardins

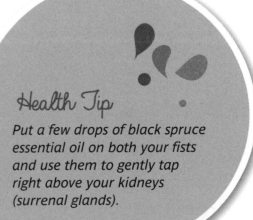

Health Tip

Put a few drops of black spruce essential oil on both your fists and use them to gently tap right above your kidneys (surrenal glands).

191

My path to well-being

Energetic cleansing consists of precisely rubbing your meridians to "purge" your body of excesses, but also to reboot it. It is advised to do it in the morning as soon as you experience stress, or in preparation of an upcoming event. Simply follow the drawing below and rub the recommended spots with your fingers. Respect what you feel. Do this while thinking about your well-being.

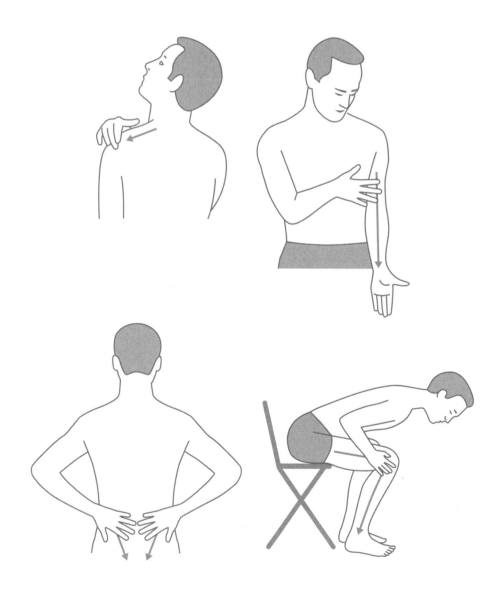

ENERGETIC POLLUTION—OTHERS' STRESS—IS A REALITY.

My cocooning space

Snacking upsets the natural functioning of the body. For those who already have an appetite, it increases the risk of putting on weight. For others, it disrupts feeling hungry or satiated. The worst are probably evening snacks. The digestion of your late intake overtaxes your system, which might disturb your sleep. These few common sense remarks will help you to remain aware and reasonable.

◎ Drink water regularly. Ingesting small quantities of water during the day decreases the feeling of hunger between meals.

◎ Establish regular feeding times. Set a time for each meal (about every four to five hours) and keep to it. Complement with a fruit or yogurt around 4 PM.

◎ Ingest fiber rich meals. Fibers take longer to digest, thus preventing you from feeling hungry too quickly.

◎ Do not skip breakfast. It should constitute 25 percent of your total daily energy intake and include whole grain bread, one fruit, and one dairy (yogurt or cheese).

◎ Eat slowly and chew your food longer to prevent stomachaches (bloating, slow digestion, etc.) and feel satiated longer.

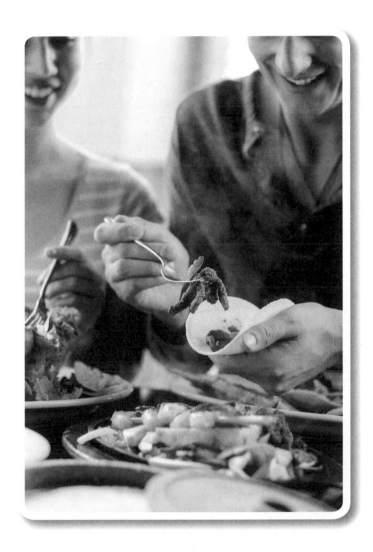

My anti-stress moment

Further working on listening to your body, we are going back to meditation and positive thinking. Take some time daily to feel compassion for your organs, for this surprising body alchemy at work since your conception, for this body that will be yours all your life, for this "realization vehicle," as Tibetans would say.

1. Sit on the edge of a chair: engage in cardiac coherence for a few moments and then name each organ you are going to "visit." For doing so, close your eyes.

2. Start with the heart. Think about smiling to your heart (for real). Bring a thought of love, visualize your regular heartbeat with enthusiasm. Then think about your lungs, feel them inflate and deflate, thank this element of life . . .

3. Bring your attention to your stomach and send some green color to regenerate it. After this, go to the pancreas, which manages your sugar and energy: think about it benevolently and visualize it in great form. Imagine that you are regenerating your intestinal flora. Turn to your liver and gallbladder, which often harbor anger. Bring them some love, calm them with tenderness and understanding, reassure them. Go up to the brain once you feel calm, balanced, and concentrated.

4. Enjoy this appeasement moment, relax, and slowly come back to the present with a big smile on your face.

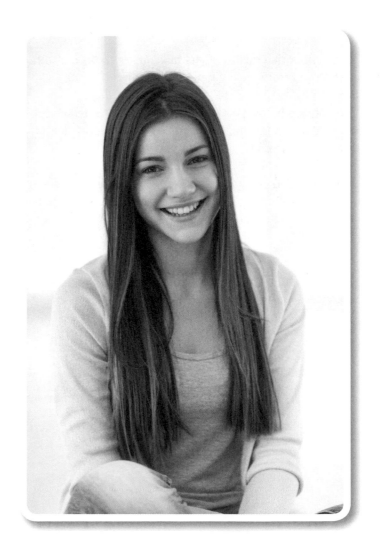

My art therapy moment

✏️ Take some space to relax

◎ Be free from dominant emotions by slowly coloring this mandala. Think about three negative emotions that are particularly problematic for you. Note them on your mandala and attribute a specific color to each one of them.

◎ In a few words, describe your need for inner free space you want to experience:

. . . .
. . . .
. . . .
. . . .
. . . .
. . . .
. . . .
. . . .
. . . .
. . . .
. . . .
. . . .
. . . .
. . . .
. . . .
. . . .

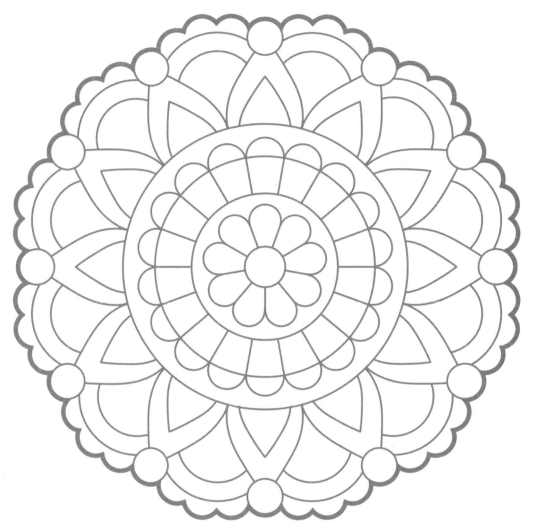

Meditate on this sentence:

Seek what you are missing in what you already have.

Zen koan

Coaching Tip

Cheer up by smiling voluntarily, sticking your tongue out of your mouth, and making circles.

My well-being path

Below is a breathing concentration set that will bring inner harmony. Be respectful, engaged in each movement. Real basic work is done slowly. It requires attention, being in the "here and now," understanding where the physical blocks, often unconscious, are located and rectifying them progressively. Then, de-stressing is immediate.

1. Think to inhale while bringing your hands up and to exhale slowly while bringing them back down.

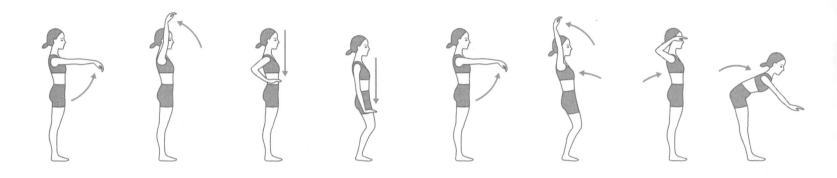

2. For this set of movements, take time to exhale fully when you are lowering your hands to your waist, at the end of the set.

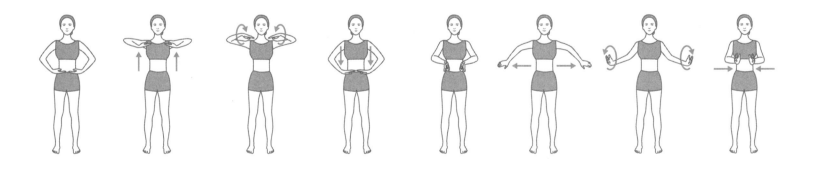

TO BE PRESENT TO MY BREATHING IS TO BE AVAILABLE TO MYSELF.

My cocooning space

Remember that pets also have their own energetic circuit and that, like you, they need harmony to live properly.

◎ Avoid setting their bed close to Wi-Fi sources.

◎ Feed them quality food, i.e. organic, not industrial.

◎ Choose competent people for their care who will not recommend products whose sources you cannot verify (useless vaccines, chemical anti-fleas, etc.)

◎ Give them well-being massages, play soothing music, and organize outdoors games.

◎ See them as evolutionary beings that need to live their experiences and their sexuality, to discover their own energetic system, their sleep rhythm . . .

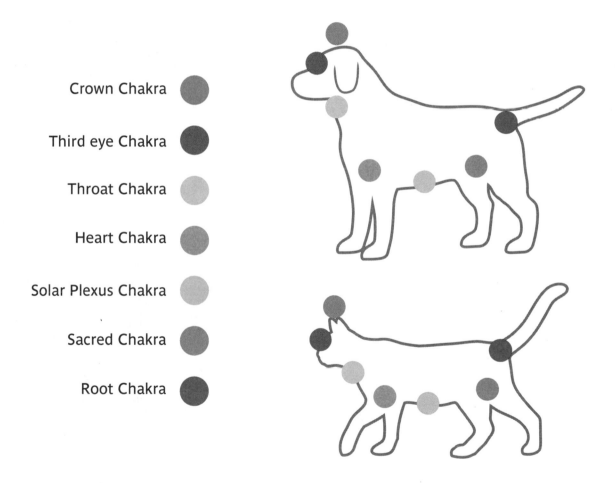

Crown Chakra

Third eye Chakra

Throat Chakra

Heart Chakra

Solar Plexus Chakra

Sacred Chakra

Root Chakra

PETS ARE SENSITIVE TO STRESS (THAT INCLUDES YOURS!)

Without knowing it, several of us practice meditative walk when we walk to relax, breathe, escape. . . . The difference here is that you are going to take the time to feel it, to enter "the art of movement." It is an interesting stress-interrupter because it forces us to act in the moment. To give more "taste" to this walk, you are going to associate a flavor to it. A most palatable activity to practice! You can take this walk during your day's work, alone, or as a family.

1. Decide on a certain course, for example, a long walk, a shorter one, or zigzagging in the streets. Looking on the ground in front of you, start to notice every movement you make. In your legs, you feel you foot going up, bringing the knee along, then your leg bending back and going forward; in turn, the hip works, the top part of your body is engaging and prepares for the other foot to go up, etc. In the same way, concentrate on your hands and arms, your torso, your back, etc. You are in the present immediately, at home, in your body.

2. Once you are familiar enough with that type of exercise, you will walk with a flavor in your mouth (a licorice stick, a zest of orange . . .) and you will feel that your mood takes on the color, the taste, and the flavor of what you have in your mouth.

3. Associate a breathing rhythm to your walk, without particularly observing all your movements. Work above all on your endurance on flat terrain: one step means one leg goes forward. Inhale on the first three paces; keep the air in your lungs on the fourth pace; exhale on the next three steps; do not breathe in during the fourth step. When you are used to this rhythm, adapt the breathing to four or five steps (without changing the ones you take in apnea and on empty lungs). You will notice that your long walks on flat terrain tire you much less.

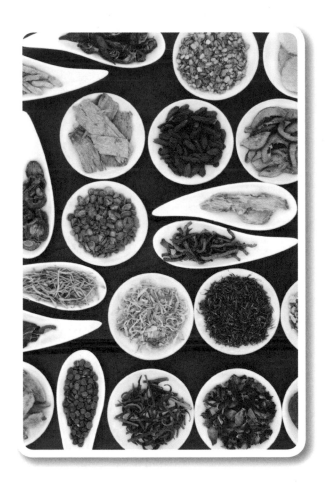

My art therapy moment

✏️ ## A sweet world

◎ Take pure pleasure in using different colors for each kitten and butterfly!

◎ Write a few words that conjure up dreams and tenderness:

....
....
....
....
....
....
....
....
....
....
....
....
....
....
....
....
....
....
....
....
....

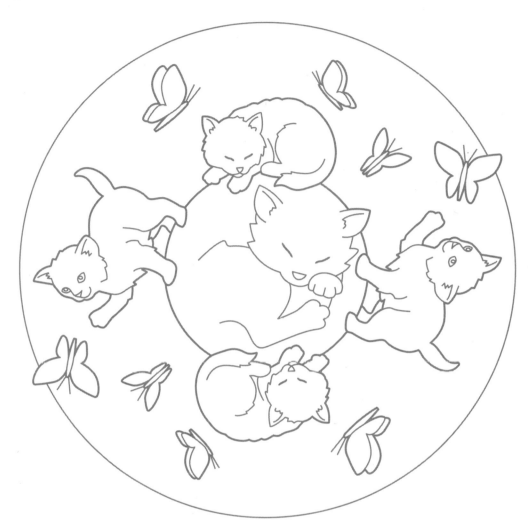

Meditate on this sentence:

To realize something truly extraordinary, dream it first.
Walt Disney

Health Tip

Take some crumpled paper or a tennis ball in your hands and play with it a few moments to relax while breathing peacefully.

My path to well-being

Breathe to live, and live better! Decide to take two minutes every morning to practice each of these exercises to cleanse from the night's toxins and start your day in great form.

Inhale   Exhale

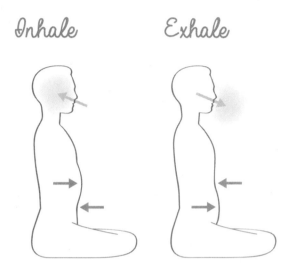

Movements and breathing coordination

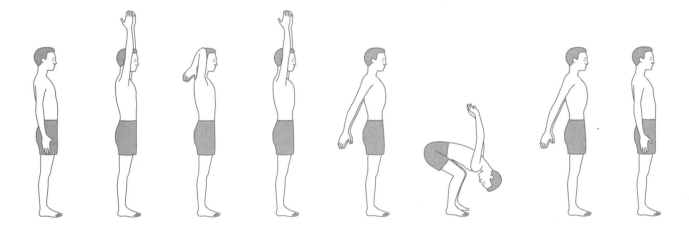

◎ Breathe in while your arms go up and behind your back. Breathe out when you bend your torso forward.

◎ Be gentle, the important thing is to empty your lungs out! Then breathe in again while standing back up.

◎ Repeat three times, being keenly aware of every movement.

My cocooning space

The health benefits and gustative qualities of spices have been known since antiquity. As other aromatic plants, spices are used to relieve or redress (as is the case, for example, in Ayurvedic medicine).

Curcuma

◎ Curcuma tea relieves colds, cough, arthritis, and toothaches. Used regularly in cooking (rice, semolina, vegetables . . .) this spice treats stomach and liver problems. Studies show that it also can prevent cancer. And it is a brain booster! A very good regulator of hormones, Curcuma also rebalances your sugar and fat cravings.

Fenugreek seeds

◎ Rich in vitamin C, potassium, fiber, protein, iron, vitamin B3, and alkaloids, these seeds can reduce LDL cholesterol, risk of stroke, and other heart diseases. They also slow down the absorption rate of sugar in the organism (which fights diabetes).

Ginger

◎ Thanks to its zingerone contents, ginger is a natural remedy against strokes because it prevents blood clot formation. It also contributes to lowering triglycerides, cholesterol, and blood pressure.

Bear's Garlic

◎ Rich in sulfur and antioxidants, bear's garlic is good for your health and your brain. It also efficiently fights cancerous cells in the brain. Use two to three cloves a day to control blood pressure and the problems it causes.

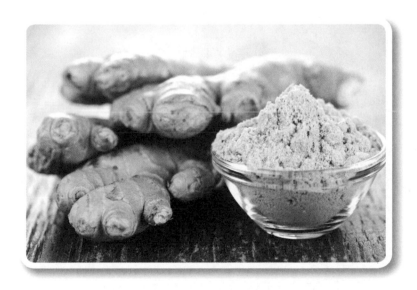

My anti-stress moment

As stress is becoming an integral part of our lives, we have no choice but using it as an agent of change. Consider this next activity a training session whose objective is to create a "reflex response" in your brain whenever stress occurs. The brain learns constantly. Learn to program it!

1. Lying down with your eyes closed, bring your attention on each point of your body. Relax . . .

2. Bring your attention on the air coming in and out of your nose.

3. Remember the place where you have lived a pleasant scene.

4. Let that memory focus on your mental screen.

5. What makes this place? What are its colors? Who are the people? Try to hear the sounds, feel the smells . . .

6. Imagine that you are touching the elements of the place, for example, the leaves, the stones. Smell their scent . . .

7. Visualize yourself serene and relaxed in that place. Use this moment to breathe calmly, feel good, peaceful, calm, recharged!

8. Now, slowly join your thumb and your index finger as if to seal the idea of well-being that you are living, the relaxation that you are experiencing, and release the pressure.

9. Slowly open your eyes and decide that each time you feel stress overtake you, you'll put your thumb and your index finger together to bring you the same calm as the one you experienced during your relaxation programming.

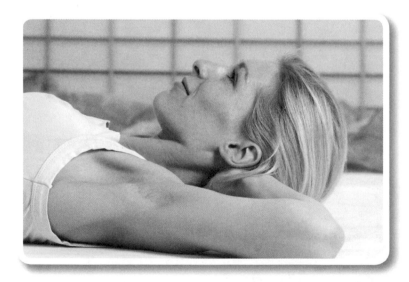

USE YOUR STRESS AS A NECESSARY ELEMENT OF CHANGE.

My art therapy moment

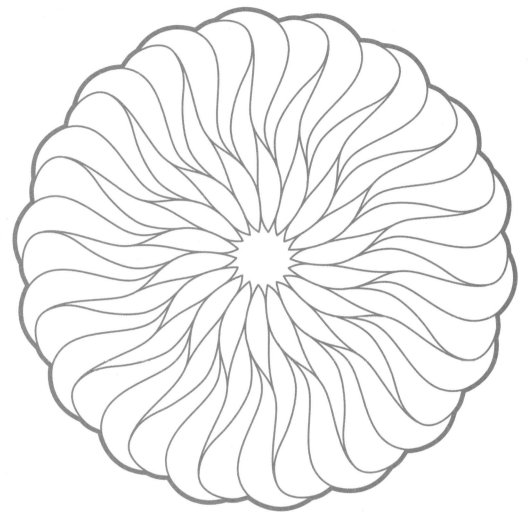

✏️ Remain serene and calm

◎ Choose colors that carry an idea of strength as well as well-being. Start from the center and progress to the exterior.

◎ Write a few words that conjure up the idea of a calm and serene strength:

....
....
....
....
....
....
....
....
....
....
....
....
....
....
....
....
....
....

Meditate on this sentence:

Man's sun is man.

Jules Michelet

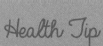

Health Tip

Standing, legs together and eyes closed, let yourself sway, from side to side, back and forth, like a culbuto. Let your center of gravity bring you up, trusting in this letting-go moment!

My path to well-being

Here is a general face massage that you can use several times a day to relax. Use your favorite facial cream during the massage to help the muscles relax. Follow the progression and the gestures!

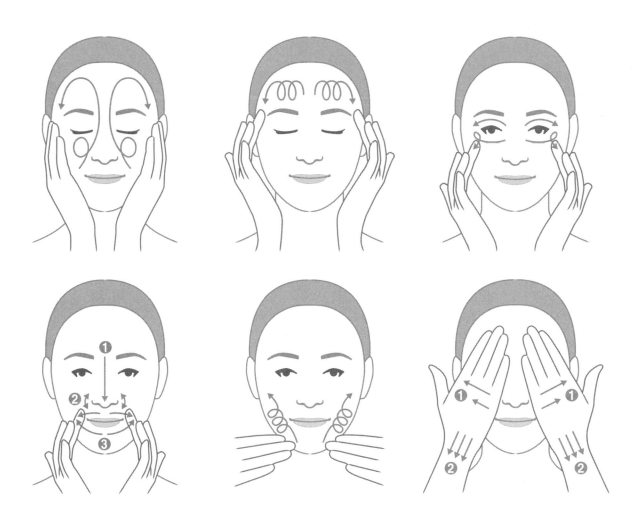

LINK BEAUTY TO ANTI-STRESS MOMENTS!

My cocooning space

 Bees' marvelous work creates subtle products used in apitherapy. Here are a few ideas to familiarize yourself with this brilliant partnership between nature and insect.

Pollens

The composition of pollens is function of the flowers from which bees have collected them. They are available fresh or frozen. The following pollens are the most commonly used in apitherapy:

◎ Cistus tree pollen contains carotenoids that protect the mucus membrane of the intestine.

◎ Willow tree pollen (harvested in the spring) contains substances that protect the retina and prevent or delay the evolution of macular degeneration caused by age.

◎ Heather pollen is recommended for blood circulation, varicose veins, and hemorrhoids. It also has a positive effect on the brain.

◎ Chestnut tree pollen, the most antioxidant, is recommended for women over forty years of age who are premenopausal because it contains phytoestrogens that slow the loss of calcium.

◎ Poppy pollen, rich in protein and vitamin C, is a perfect accompaniment to a vegetarian regimen.

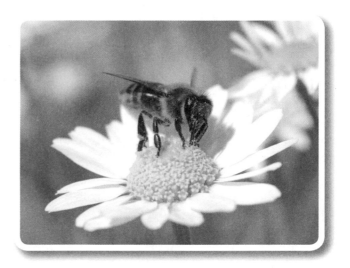

Propolis

◎ Propolis is a rare natural antibiotic that bees harvest on tree buds and store on their hind legs to bring back to the beehive.

Royal jelly

◎ This milky substance is secreted by the glands of feeding bees. It is a choice food in the hive since only the queen bee feeds on it its whole life. Royal jelly reduces cholesterol and strengthens the immunity system.

HONEY AND POLLEN ARE NATURALLY RICH IN NUTRIENTS.

Anti-stress "presence" Test

One of the basics of anti-stress is to be able to react serenely and instantly. Here are two simple tests that you have to memorize for each period of your day. You need to be attentive to what you experience but also to what your body uses as an alert message. We are talking about two different types of listening and meditative attentions here; do not hesitate to use them each week. We have left some space so you can write the other recurring stressors that you experience.

1. Personalize the exercise by answering the question at a key moment; rectify if necessary by investing more awareness in the moment. This means being conscious of movement, being in the thought corresponding to the activity experienced.

Am I really present in my body? Am I in the thought that corresponds with the activity experienced?

◎ While taking my morning shower
◎ During my breakfast
◎ During my morning commute
◎ During my morning activities or workday
◎ When I listen to colleagues or family telling me the same story again and again
◎ When I have to make decisions and back them up
◎ When I need to stay calm and constructive
◎ When finally I have lunch quietly without having to take anybody's stress on my shoulders
◎ When I hear good or bad news
◎ When I learn I need to modify my weekend plans
◎ While assessing what I have to do before the end of the day
◎ Leaving work or closing the door on the day's activities
◎ Coming back to my loved ones
◎ Imagining the evening to come
◎ Forcing myself to take a relaxing moment before going on to the next activity
◎ Lying down and concentrating on my wish for a peaceful night

◎ Other topics of attention:

....
....
....
....
....
....
....
....
....

2. Scan the drawing of the body below. Sit down, take time to breathe slowly, and put your attention on each point from head to toe, your breath bringing your wish to relax the painful points. Then, note in red (each week) the points that are still painful or bruised. Keep your drawings and compare, month after month, the recurring painful points. Think about correcting your posture every day, about possibly consulting an osteopath, and/or about signing up for yoga classes or a non-violent sport! A naturopath can also suggest a physical well-being regimen. The important point is to become aware and act accordingly during the year!

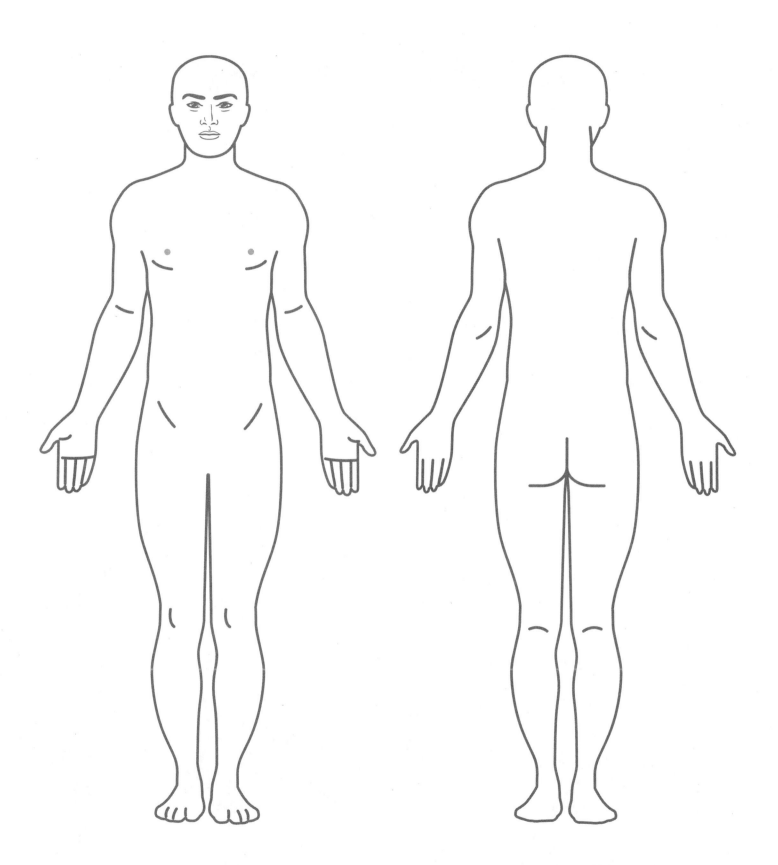